2538.

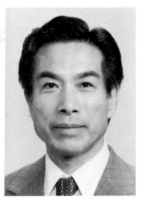

Professor Hikaru Hamano is famous in Japan and the United States as a foremost expert on the use of contact lenses and he is head of a large group of ophthalmologists where contact lenses are prescribed.

He is Assistant Professor at Osaka University Medical School and Visiting Professor at Louisiana State University School of Medicine. He is the author of over 150 research papers and books. Professor Hamano is Director of the Japan Contact Lens Council and Contact Lens Society and editor of the Society's Journal

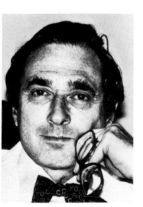

Professor Montague Ruben FRCS, LRCP, DOMS is Consultant Ophthalmologist and former director of the Department of Contact Lenses and Prosthetics at Moorfield's Eye Hospital in London, and Visiting Professor at the Ophthalmic and Optic Department at the City University, London. He is the author of *A Textbook on Contact Lens Practice, Understanding Contact Lenses, Soft Contact Lens Practice* and the *Illustrated Atlas of Contact Lenses.*

Professor Ruben has recently taken up an appointment as Director of the Institute for Contact Lens Research at the University of Houston, Texas.

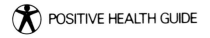
POSITIVE HEALTH GUIDE

CONTACT LENSES
A guide to successful wear and care

Professor Hikaru Hamano
and
Professor Montague Ruben, FRCS, LRCP, DOMS

MARTIN DUNITZ

© Hikaru Hamano and Montague Ruben 1985

First published in the United Kingdom in 1985
by Martin Dunitz Ltd, 154 Camden High Street, London NW1 0NE

Reprinted 1986

British Library Cataloguing in Publication Data

Ruben, Montague
 Contact lenses: a guide to successful wear and care. – (Positive health guide).
 1. Contact lenses
 I. Title II. Hamano, Hikaru III. Series
 617.7'523 RE977.C6

ISBN 0-906348-87-0
ISBN 0-906348-88-9 Pbk

Phototypeset by Book Ens, Saffron Walden, Essex
Printed by Toppan Printing Company (S) Pte Ltd, Singapore

CONTENTS

INTRODUCTION

Contact lenses are among the most useful aids to seeing. A great many people with near or far sight, or with astigmatism, don't want either the discomfort or change to their looks that results from wearing glasses. Others, who have surgery for a cataract, can (if they haven't had a lens implant) have their sight perfectly restored by contact lenses. For these people lenses are ideal. Once anyone has adjusted to putting them in and wearing them for long periods, the advantages of better sight without the bother of glasses far outweigh the time and effort needed to adapt.

If you have the choice between wearing contact lenses and glasses you will want to know about their relative benefits and disadvantages. This book should help you make up your mind as to whether you will be suited to using contact lenses. If you have already decided you want them, we tell you how to get the best from wearing them – by treating both the lenses and your eyes correctly.

With so many types of lenses made from hundreds of different plastics, and of varying hardness or softness, you may be uncertain which type you are being offered and why. We explain why you are likely to be prescribed a particular sort and how long you should be able to go on wearing your lenses before they need replacing.

We have recognized the need for a book such as this just because there are so many contact lens wearers and potential wearers. The book's usefulness has already been shown by its great success in Japan. It was originally written by Dr Hikaru Hamano for his patients there and it was exceedingly popular. He wanted English-speaking people to have the benefit of the advice and explanations. When asked to see a literal translation, Professor Montague Ruben realized that a better way to convey the essence of the book was to rewrite and illustrate as necessary, and so the present book is not a translation but a new one on the same subject.

1 HOW DOES THE EYE WORK?

Before understanding how contact lenses help poor vision, you need to know how the eye works and what may go wrong with normal sight that can be helped by wearing lenses.

The anatomy of the eye

The simplest way of understanding how the eye works is to think of it as a camera. The lens at the front receives the picture and transmits it to a film at the back of the eye (the retina). That picture is continually being printed in the brain by the messages sent along a nerve pipeline joining the eye to the brain (the optic nerve). The picture actually arrives on the retina upside down – as in a camera – but the brain perceives the image the right way up.

The same process is happening in both eyes. Each has a different field of vision on the outer edges, but the brain also joins together what is seen to make one three dimensional picture – stereoscopic vision.

The pupil
If you look at your eye in a mirror you see the white (sclera), the black pupil and the coloured iris. If you look carefully and the light is good you may also notice a very small picture of yourself formed in the pupil; that is why it is called the pupil – a small person. The reason you can see this is that you are reflected from the transparent coating called the cornea that covers the central part of the eye. The light entering the eye is regulated by the pupil acting like the aperture on a camera. The iris muscles close the pupil to bright light, and in dim light it is opened up to make a large aperture – so that the coloured iris becomes a narrower rim.

The retina
The retina is the layer covering the inside of the eyeball; it consists of many hundreds of thousands of light-sensitive cells. There are two types, rods and cones, so-called because of their shapes. The majority, the rods, are concerned only with receiving crude messages, not detailed pictures; they can adapt to both night and daytime vision. But concentrated into an area no bigger than the size of a pinhead (the

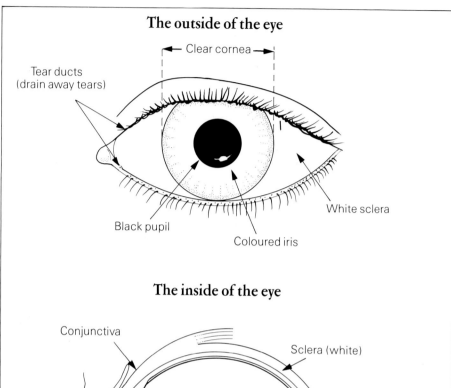

The outside of the eye

Clear cornea

Tear ducts
(drain away tears)

White sclera

Black pupil

Coloured iris

The inside of the eye

Conjunctiva

Sclera (white)

Ciliary muscle

Cornea
Pupil
Aqueous
humour (fluid)

Iris

L
E
N
S

Vitreous humour
(fluid)

Optic nerve

Retina (light sensitive)

Choroid (blood vessels)

The anatomy of the eye.

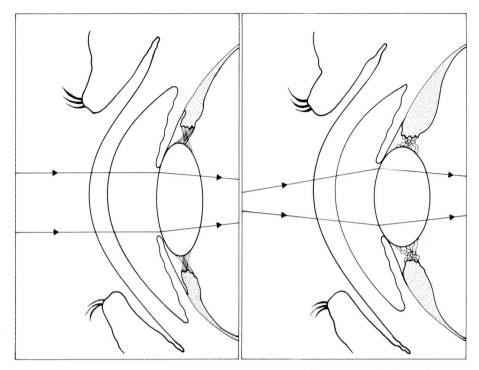

The ciliary muscle adjusts the position of the lens for near or far focusing.

macula) there are several thousand cells, the cones, that specialize in daytime colour vision and fine detail. It is these cells that bring the object you are looking at into sharp focus. The diagram above shows how the eye focuses; a contact lens used to correct vision has to simulate the eye lens as far as possible.

The cornea

This is a very important part of the eye from our point of view, since it is on the cornea itself that the contact lens is fitted.

Imagine the cornea magnified a thousand times. First, covering it, is the tear film, which keeps the cornea transparent. Beneath the tear film lies the cornea itself, consisting of several layers of cells. These surface cells die if the tear film dries, making the cornea opaque. Underneath them there is a thick section of fibres and finally a layer of thin cells. The fascinating thing is that the cornea, although made up of all these cells and fibres, is still almost 100 per cent transparent.

The tear film   Like the oil in your motor car, tears have a lubricant function, but they also affect your sight and have a nutritional role. It

11

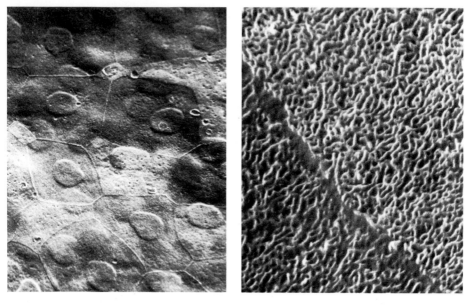

Above The corneal surface of a rabbit's eye (very similar to a human's) seen through an electron microscope. *Left* The regularly arranged cells are clearly visible, and, *right*, higher magnification shows the wrinkled projections the tears cling to.

Below The layers of the tear film.

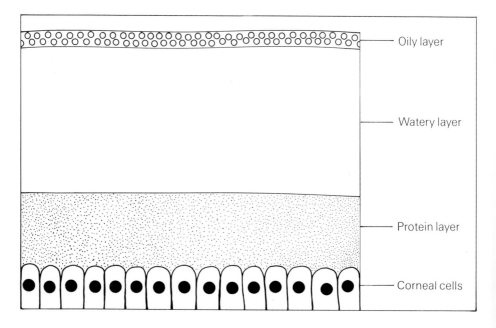

does seem amazing that a film of fluid no more that a fraction of a millimetre thick has so many functions. It can do all these things because tears are not just one fluid like water but made up of several parts:

1. The watery tears are formed by a gland under the lid. As we blink, the eyeball is washed by fresh tears made up of water and natural salts. They drain away through the drainage channel. Whenever we cry emotionally or from eye irritation the tear gland works overtime and produces an excess of tears that cannot all drain away and so spill over on to our cheeks. In the same way the glands in the mouth produce juices when stimulated by food or smells.

   While some tears help, too many can affect the vision and even the transparency of the eye tissue. If you cry a lot or put solutions, perhaps eyedrops, in your eyes that have a different saline content from tears, the cells on the surface of the cornea tend to separate and may even swell up, giving hazy vision. People who have cried a lot often find their vision is blurred. The same reaction can occur from wearing contact lenses that produce too many tears (see also Chapter 6).

2. As well as the water and salts there is a protein part to the tears. Rather like the transparent part of the egg that surrounds the yolk, there are similar substances that cover the white of the eye and under-surface of the lids. This sticky substance forms a deeper layer mixed with the tears.

3. Floating on top of the protein solution is a thin layer of oil, which comes from the glands that are situated along the lids (see the diagram on page 10). This is smeared over the eye by the edges of the eyelids, and prevents the watery tears from evaporating.

The first layer, the tears, keeps the eye moist and free of dust, while the second and third protect and feed it. The oily layer is the one that is often affected by the contact lens, and as we shall see in Chapter 5 it is the protein and oil of the tears that can spoil the surface of the lens.

You might wonder how the tear film stays on the front of the eye. Part of the answer is it is so very thin that it clings to the eyeball. There are also very fine microscopic fingers on the cells of the cornea and these may hold the sticky layer of the tears in place.

Why are tears so important?   Tears are produced to wash and protect the eye. They wash away bacteria and foreign particles that may enter the eye. They also contain special enzymes that can destroy harmful bacteria. Although the supply of tears is constant it can suddenly be increased by dryness on the front of the eye or anything that causes irritation of the eye.

Your contact lens will touch the front of the eye all day, maybe sometimes night and day for several days, months or even years, depending on the type you have, and the eye should not be affected in any way. With good, plentiful tears and a clear, transparent cornea you will be able to wear contact lenses. The pictures on page 12 show the surface of the corneal tear film magnified. The irregularities and dry areas show a cornea that would be unsuitable for contact lens wear (see also Chapter 6 on pregnancy).

How the cornea is nourished and breathes All the body tissues receive food in the form of intricate chemicals via the bloodstream. One of these used by the body to make energy is glucose. It is a simple sugar that the body makes from the food taken in. Besides the nourishment from the tear film (see above) the small cells of the cornea need this glucose night and day. Although there are no blood vessels in the cornea, the glucose is absorbed from the liquids in the eye and the tears. Glucose is stored in the cells of the cornea as glycogen and is used whenever the normal supply is used up. A contact lens that does not allow the eye to breathe can interfere with this (see Chapter 3).

The blood and tears also bring oxygen to the cells and take away gases that are formed as they burn up energy. This cycle is like burning coal or oil in a stove to produce hot water. The coal requires oxygen from the air to burn and produce heat. When burning, the fuel produces gases which are taken away by the flue. In the same way the cornea gets its oxygen from both the atmosphere and the blood. This is important for contact lens wearers because the cornea must stay clear and not become spoilt through poor ventilation (see Chapter 6). Bad contact lenses or even good contact lenses badly worn can spoil this front window.

The eye is a delicate instrument and its focusing power can be affected in a number of ways so that artificial lenses, whether in glasses or as contact lenses, are necessary to readjust the focusing back to normal. In the next chapter we describe those focusing problems and the ways they are put right.

2 WHICH EYE PROBLEMS ARE TREATED WITH CONTACT LENSES?

We have seen that the most important part of the eye for contact lens wearers is the pupil covered by the clear cornea. The functions that can be corrected by lenses are mainly problems of focusing. The commonest are near sight (myopia), far sight (hypermetropia or hypertropia), astigmatism, unequal sighted eyes, loss of near focus (presbyopia) and a lazy eye (strabismus or squint).

Near sight (myopia)

This can occur from birth but is usually discovered in young children, when they start school and complain of not seeing very well in class, or during the teenage years when there is extra studying for examinations. It is a defect of growth and does not often go undetected into old age.

Near sight is a very common condition affecting between 10 and 15 per cent of the sixteen to eighteen age group. It is slightly more common in Asiatics than in Caucasian whites and may be hereditary. It often develops over a period of a year but in that time you probably won't realize you have become near-sighted. You do not lose the ability to focus on near objects but when looking at anything over about 3 feet (1 metre) it becomes blurred. Near sight is easily corrected by glasses or contact lenses.

What has happened can again be explained by thinking of the eye as a camera. The eye has grown too long and so the clear image is formed in front of the retina (see diagram overleaf). If you were using a camera it would be as if the lens were set for a near focus and then the picture taken of a distant object. A clear picture would be obtained by adjusting the lens of the camera so that it would be farther away from the film. When the eye becomes too long for the lens it is impossible to move the lens farther away from the retina, but we can weaken the power of the eye by wearing glasses or contact lenses that move the point of focus back in the eye.

Glasses or contact lenses?
The spectacle lens makes the picture formed at the back of the eye bright and smaller than normal, and providing the power is not too high

there is very little distortion. With glasses, however, the sight is corrected in one position and we get used to making allowances for the changes in vision as the eyes move. People with very near sight must wear thick glasses, and these create quite a lot of distortion (see page 28). This effect is reduced by making the area of the glasses lens you look through small. Although this helps, it has the bad effect of restricting or distorting vision from the sides and below. In this case especially, glasses become both an optical and physical encumbrance, and many people decide to try contact lenses to correct their near sight, or sometimes they even have operations.

The contact lens has certain benefits over glasses in correcting near sight. Because the contact lens is placed right on the eye your sight is corrected wherever it moves. The image formed at the back of the eye is also larger and this is especially helpful if you are very near-sighted. But the lens may not be the perfect solution:

1. Unless of special design, it can make things worse if you have poor focusing ability for close work – especially if the lens is too strong;

2. If you started with glasses, your eyes will have learnt to work with

Near sight: the image formed in front of the retina, and *right*, corrected by a concave lens.

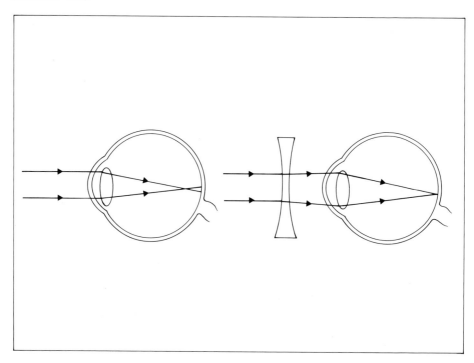

them; they will have to learn again with contact lenses, particularly for close work, as the way the lens corrects near sight is different from glasses (see page 29).

This difficulty with close vision can make contact lenses a disadvantage, especially for people from their early forties onwards. If they are not very near-sighted they can wear glasses for distance vision and for close vision take them off and have perfect sight (see page 20). Contact lenses can't be so easily put in and removed.

As close sight is not a problem for someone who is middle-aged and near-sighted, contact lenses, especially strong ones, will mean glasses have to be worn for reading. The choice is between glasses for distance, or contact lenses, with glasses for reading. The very near-sighted have little to lose and a lot to gain by changing to contact lenses. They will have better distance and all-round vision. For the middle-aged, on balance, the use of additional reading glasses is a small price to pay for the advantages. The future will undoubtedly see contact lenses that in the age groups over forty help both distance and close vision (see Chapter 7).

Although contact lenses are usually the best solution for near-sighted people, they are not always right for near-sighted children. In Mary's case, it took a lot of discussion with specialists to decide whether she would be able to wear contact lenses successfully:

When she was eight years old, Mary brought home from school a piece of paper. The note said that the school nurse had tested her vision and that the result was not satisfactory. An appointment would soon be made with the local eye specialist. The examination was a week later and showed that Mary was near-sighted. While able to read the smallest print when held close, she was unable to see large letters at even 10 feet (3 metres).

Mary's parents were not surprised to find that one of their three children had developed near sight as both of them had been near-sighted since their teens. Mary's mother had worn contact lenses from the age of sixteen and her father had had glasses since he was eleven. He had tried contact lenses once but could not adapt to them. He was told that because of an allergic skin condition and bad hay fever he should stick to glasses.

Mary's mother asked the eye doctor about all the modern treatments for near sight. Unfortunately the doctor was rather severe and answered curtly that only glasses were advised and that was all there was to it. When Mary's mother persisted the doctor rudely said, 'The trouble with all these women's magazines is that they think modern science can cure everything!'

This attitude upset Mary's mother, who worried about having

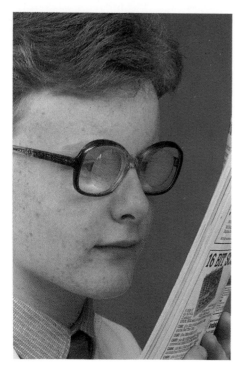

People with poor sight may need thick spectacle lenses. Sometimes better vision is possible with special low vision aids which magnify and are set in the spectacle frame. For people with very short sight, contact lenses also act as magnifiers.

spoiled her daughter's life because of this inherited sight problem. She worried her husband and they eventually both went to see another eye doctor to discuss what they could do. Should Mary wear the glasses the first doctor had prescribed or not? They were convinced from their own experience that once you started wearing glasses that was the end, and every year the glasses became stronger until you were blind as a bat without them. They considered glasses as an invention of opticians to stop people getting better sight! The eye doctor realized after an hour that the same questions with variations were being asked again and again and no progress was being made. So he suggested they take Mary to a famous ophthalmologist in the city, who was well known for his views on whether children could wear contact lenses. They should let him be the final arbiter.

The ophthalmologist explained that short sight could in some cases be temporary and induced by increased close work. More often it was due to the eye growing longer than it should. After all, you couldn't expect every eye to grow exactly to within a millimetre of its correct size. In any event, he would do a few simple tests, including

18

the use of drops to relax the eye's muscle that allows accommodation (reading focus). Then he would be able to give a proper diagnosis. He explained that some of his special instruments could electronically even measure the length of the eye.

Unfortunately Mary's near sight was due to the eye being too long and an operation could not help at her age. The ophthalmologist advised glasses now but of a design that would not cause further development of near sight, and then later on contact lenses. The contact lenses would give Mary more confidence and better all-round vision, providing her eye tissue accepted them, and she would eventually learn how to manage them herself. He suggested the age of twelve would be a good time to start.

Eventually Mary was fitted with soft lenses for one year. She then changed to hard, gas permeable, corneal ones, since she had developed a little astigmatism which was best corrected by this type of lens. Fifteen years later Mary will still be wearing lenses all day and every day, except most of Sunday when she will give her eyes a well-earned rest.

Far sight: the image formed behind the retina, and *right*, corrected by a convex lens.

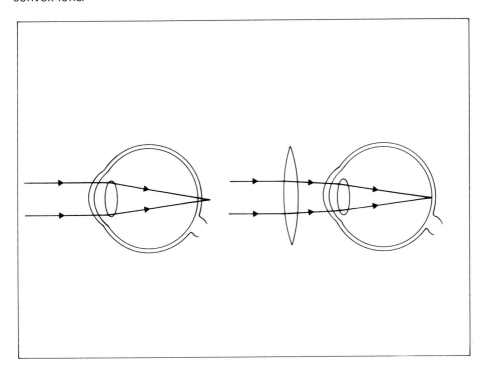

Far sight (hypertropia)

This is the opposite of near sight and, although common enough, is far less common than near sight; about 5 per cent of the population in the sixteen to eighteen age group is far-sighted. Like close sight, it may be an inherited condition. The eye is too short so that the point of focus is behind the retina and the image cannot be formed clearly. The far-sighted eye can adjust the power by accommodation of the lens of the eye so that light entering the eye from the distance can be brought to a focus on the retina. But there is a limit to how much adjusting it can do. Young children have great powers of adjustment but after the age of twenty this gradually diminishes. Uncorrected large degrees of far sight are in any case bad for the long term. Even if a child can drastically change the eye power it is not possible for both eyes to work together while this is happening. Too much far sight without optical correction can lead to one eye becoming less used than the other and even the development of a lazy eye, that can turn in or out of true (see page 27).

Glasses or lenses?

Children and adults alike resent wearing glasses to correct small degrees of far sight since they see equally well with and without glasses. It is only for close work that spectacles are a must. Contact lenses are therefore a great boon, especially for children, if they are combined with treatment to correct lazy eyes (see page 27).

Loss of close vision (presbyopia)

The eyes have to alter their focus to change from looking into the distance to looking at near objects (see the diagram opposite). The additional plus power necessary to do this is called accommodation. The lens in the eye becomes rounder and so of stronger power. After the age of forty there is a gradual loss of this faculty. Losing close vision, which happens to everyone, is called presbyopia. To begin with, loss of a little power is barely noticeable. You can correct it just by holding reading matter a little further away. But after a time the book or paper has to be held too far from the eyes for the print to be readable, even if in focus. At this point you realize you can't do without glasses any longer so either you go to the optometrist or you borrow someone else's reading glasses. Many people, and especially in places where expert eye testing is not available, buy reading glasses over the counter. These are usually graded in a few powers according to age. They are not likely to do you any harm unless you choose very strong ones. These will cause discomfort and rapidly increase the need for stronger and stronger glasses.

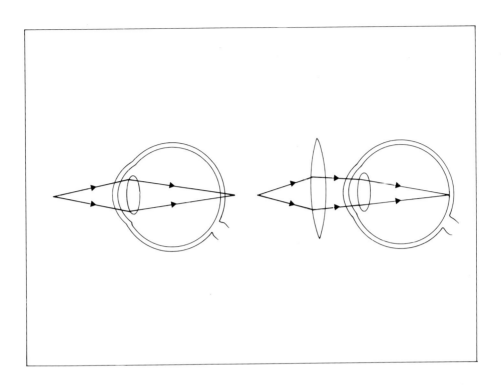

Presbyopia: close vision is brought back into focus with a convex lens.

Glasses or lenses?

People with loss of close vision (presbyopia) always ask whether contact lenses can be prescribed. If you are already wearing them to correct another condition, over the age of forty you will still lose the power of accommodation and need reading glasses. In fact, near-sighted people wearing contact lenses who insist on wearing the full or over-all strength powers may begin to lose close vision before the age of forty. Contact lenses, usually the hard type, can be made with more than one power, or combinations of contact lenses and glasses can be worn; but the perfect contact lens to correct distance vision and presbyopia has yet to be made (see Chapter 7). In the meantime glasses alone are more satisfactory.

Astigmatism

The cornea is almost spherical at the centre but if you can imagine a vertical and horizontal line drawn across the whole cornea, you find in most people the vertical line has a steeper curve than the horizontal.

This is most likely due to the eyelid muscles moulding the cornea to that shape. The shape of the curvatures are very different in some people. This is the commonest cause of astigmatism. The lens itself can also be distorted and cause astigmatism, but of a lesser degree. Because of the distortion the light rays enter the eye at an angle of less than 90 degrees to each other, so part of the image is not formed on the retina (see the diagram below). This results in blurred vision.

About 50 per cent of people with near or far sight have astigmatism. In most cases it is a condition you are born with, and may be inherited. Glasses can correct most degrees of it but if it is irregular, this is not possible. Irregular astigmatism occurs mostly after eye disease or surgical operations and is much less common.

Glasses or lenses?

The contact lens corrects astigmatism in a different way from glasses. A hard contact lens placed on the eye does not change its shape and the space between it and the cornea is filled with tear fluid. The tear fluid and the front of the cornea are almost of the same nature so optically speaking they merge while the contact lens becomes the false and

Astigmatism: light rays enter the eye at different angles and form a blurred image.

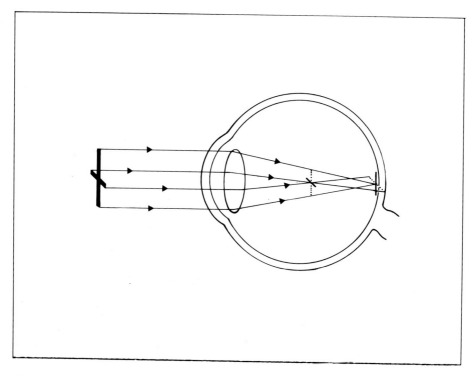

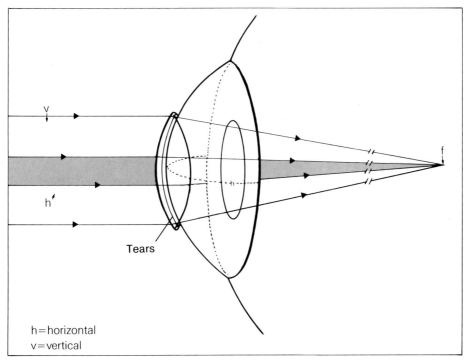

V
↓
h′

Tears

h = horizontal
v = vertical

f

A hard corneal lens is spherical and the astigmatic cornea now has no power because the tears behind the lens have the same refractive quality as the cornea. So the new front of the eye optically is the contact lens.

perfect cornea of the eye. A soft contact lens will mould to the shape of the cornea and so cannot correct astigmatism in this way, but when a soft lens is necessary for comfort, correcting power can be introduced that almost fully corrects the astigmatism. The lenses with this special correcting power are called toric lenses and are described more fully in Chapter 7.

For most people with astigmatism one or other type of lens is an ideal way of correcting the problem. But there are cases when the astigmatism is not corrected by either of these methods. In eyes without obvious astigmatism the contact lens can bring it out. If the degree of astigmatism is slight it is undetected. But when a contact lens is fitted a greater, and obvious, astigmatism is produced.

Fortunately this happens very rarely, but when it does, it can be a great source of frustration, both to the person wanting lenses and the specialist. The wearer asks, 'Why can I see perfectly with glasses but not so well with contact lenses?' Regrettably, contact lens wear has to be abandoned when hidden astigmatism that cannot be corrected with toric lenses is revealed.

23

Unequal vision

Most people – probably 85 per cent of the population – have very nearly the same vision with both eyes. One is usually more dominant than the other but when tested the difference between them is hardly noticeable. In fact, we see as with one eye (see below) and it is only when something actually goes wrong with one eye that the confusion or interference becomes obvious.

1. The usual cause of unequal vision is periods of rapid body growth, when one eye may become very different from the other.

2. More rarely, one eye may be abnormal from birth.

3. After operations on the eye or injuries the affected eye may end up different from the normal eye.

Each eye has a slightly different field of vision, but normally the brain can join these together to form a single picture.

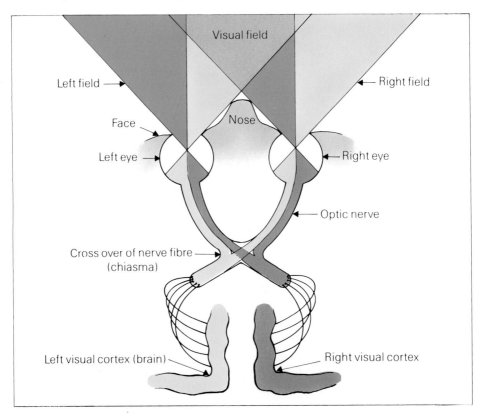

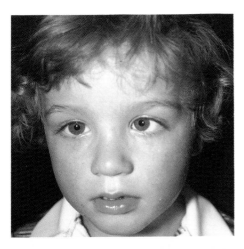

A young boy with a convergent strabismus.

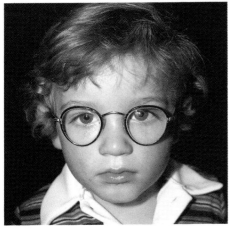

The strabismus is corrected with glasses fitted with lenses of suitable powers (see page 27).

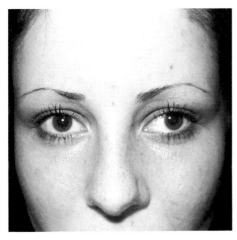

A divergent strabismus, with the left eye looking outwards.

When people have unequal vision, they naturally use the better eye most of the time, the other only occasionally. An example of unequal vision would be when one eye is far-sighted and the other is near-sighted. When this is corrected with glasses the result can be one eye seeing objects bigger than the other, leading to confusion and even the inability to use both eyes together. Contact lenses reduce this problem to a minimum. Because they can correct the weaker eye, bringing about more normal sight than glasses without distorting objects, they can be of great help. When unequal vision is caused by 1 or 2 above, fitting a suitable lens to the weaker eye helps vision immediately and avoids a lazy eye developing later. In time equal vision can be restored.

When lenses are not suitable
People requiring urgent treatment for unequal vision because their sight is very poor, or because of injury, may not be suitable for lenses: perhaps they are not easy to fit, or because of the nature of the injury there is a great time lapse from onset to diagnosis and treatment. The brain may have forgotten how to use both eyes together, or it may never have learnt; even with good will and tolerance of a contact lens, it is sometimes not possible to achieve vision for the affected eye. More exasperating still, you may be able to get good vision in both eyes with lenses and yet they cannot work together.

What can be done in these cases? It is not just a matter of fitting the correct power contact lens in the hope of arriving at an acceptable compromise. The weaker eye has to be encouraged and this may involve several hours of exercising it, with the good eye covered up. It may mean wearing contact lenses on both eyes even though the better eye may have normal sight. Then again, achieving a balance between the two eyes that produces stereoscopic vision may mean having to wear glasses and contact lenses together. By using both it is possible to correct magnification and position of the image at the same time. The use of glasses or contact lenses alone does not achieve the same result. The specialist may use as well various light stimulations to encourage the poor-sighted eye to fix upon objects.

The idea of glasses plus contact lenses to help undeveloped sight in one eye can be difficult to accept. It is used only in special cases and does not apply to the normal range of eye defects. But you shouldn't resist the idea if it is suggested for you. At best you will have good vision restored; at worst, the level of vision will be improved.

Strabismus (lazy eye or squint)

You normally have stereoscopic vision because of the sensitive nervous system that keeps the images perceived from each eye joined within narrow limits. When you look at very close objects, your eyes are unable to converge and still maintain single vision. If the object is too near, your eyes cross, leaving one eye to keep the near object in view (think of looking at the tip of your nose with both eyes). If one eye is stronger than the other this sensitive system can be put out.

The weaker eye is not properly controlled by the eye muscles and wanders, looking too far outwards (divergent strabismus) or inwards (convergent strabismus). This is by far the most commonplace eye problem in children, usually noticed when a baby first starts to focus on objects or when a child begins school. It is important to have strabismus put right before the age of eight, as after this little can be done to improve the lazy eye. There are three ways that strabismus may be corrected:

1. With glasses or contact lenses
2. By patching
3. By operation.

Many lazy eyes are put right by the first method. If this doesn't work a patch is put over the stronger eye to make the weaker one work harder. Probably one third of lazy eyes are corrected by a combination of these two methods. When neither treatment corrects the strabismus an operation on the eye muscles will bring the lazy eye to the proper position.

In most cases strabismus that can be put right by glasses can also be treated by contact lenses. Lenses of the correct powers are fitted to each eye to produce best normal vision, so teaching the lazy eye to work properly. When the lazy eye starts to do this, the lenses can sometimes be left off. The advantage of contact lenses is that children with strabismus will probably prefer them to glasses and be more likely to wear them continuously (see also Chapter 4).

When are contact lenses not effective?

Glasses have their power at a distance from the eyeball and the eye looks through different portions of the lens. This can help strabismus. The reason is that the spectacle lenses have a prism effect, while most contact lenses (except the scleral or haptic types – see Chapter 3) do not have controlled prism powers.

Glasses or contact lenses?

The choice between them depends on what sight problem you have and probably too its degree. This chapter has described the conditions where contact lenses would be appropriate. To help you make your final decision we sum up here the advantages and disadvantages of contact lenses compared with glasses:

1. Distortion

In glasses the lenses vary in thickness, depending on the weakness of vision. The shape of the glasses lens creates distortion and the thicker the glass the greater this is. The eye, looking through the centre and then suddenly switching to the edge, sees the object being looked at move. This is called a prism effect.

If you look through a prism you can see how a straight line becomes bent (see the diagram below). Even though the prism effect is gradual as the eye moves across the glasses lens and does not disturb the wearer very much, it can be a nuisance. This distortion can also affect stereoscopic vision (or simultaneous vision – see page 24) until the brain has had time to compensate.

Big lenses, which are often worn as fashion glasses, also have a

The prism effect: light rays bend and cause distortion as the eye moves.

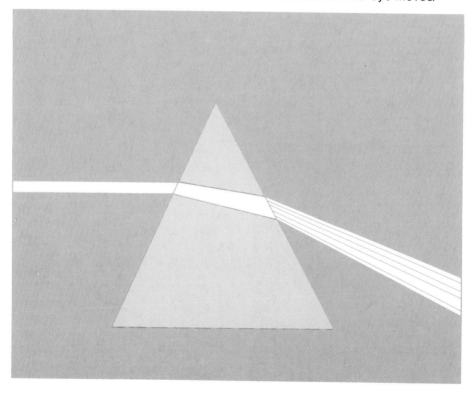

distorting effect, so doors can appear to be on a slant and ceilings not quite true.

Contact lenses do have these effects, but to a lesser degree. For anyone needing high-powered correction, wearing contact lenses should be a real advantage.

2. Lens strength
Because of its closeness to the pupil, the contact lens often does not need to be as strong as the glasses. The image formed at the back of the eye for the near-sighted is larger and less dazzling than with glasses – an effect which makes many near-sighted people who wear spectacles choose lenses weaker than their full prescription, so they may not see well.

For far-sighted people the image is smaller than with glasses. The power needed for contact lenses can be greater than for glasses. However, when far sight is fully corrected by contact lenses close work is easier than with glasses because the wearer does not have to accommodate so much.

3. Eye problems
Some can be treated only by contact lenses. These are: extreme far and near sight, unequal vision and astigmatism. People with keratoconus (a cone-shaped cornea) or who have had a cataract operation are often better off with a contact lens (see Chapter 8).

4. Cosmetic effect
This is the major reason for many people trying contact lenses. Either they feel glasses don't look good, or they find them heavy and uncomfortable. The freedom of contact lenses is worth the effort involved in getting used to them.

5. Comfort
To start with, wearing contact lenses is certainly more uncomfortable than glasses. In the long term, provided you can learn to adapt, you don't notice you're wearing them. Glasses, on the other hand, may be heavy on the bridge of the nose, steamy or sticky in wet or hot weather.

There are, though, some common eye conditions that make wearing contact lenses impossible:

Dry eyes If your tear glands don't make enough tears your eyes become gritty and sore. The discomfort is relieved with eyedrops and by avoiding a dry or rapidly ventilated atmosphere. But contact lenses would irritate the soreness and so are unsuitable.

Wet eyes   As explained in Chapter 1, too many tears interfere with your vision. Watering eyes may be due to a cold, a foreign body or crying. But if your eyes are continually watery, this may be due to a blockage in the drainage channels and until it has been put right it will not be possible to wear contact lenses.

6. Adapting to lenses
It takes some perseverance to get used to lenses and a lot of people give up in the first two or three weeks. Motivation is of course all important. In Chapter 5 we also give practical advice on how to adjust gradually and successfully to your lenses.

7. Expense
The cost of contact lenses is generally higher than a pair of fashion glasses (depending of course on the glasses chosen – high fashion glasses can cost far more than contact lenses). In the English speaking world, where this book is likely to be read, there are different types of eye health care systems. For example, in the UK patients can have a free eye test paid for by the National Health Service, but contact lenses have to be paid for unless they are medically advised and authorized by a hospital ophthalmologist. In Australia the state pays a very handsome contribution towards examination fees and the cost of the lenses, whereas in North America a totally different system exists. There eye physicians (ophthalmologists) and eye doctors (optometrists) all offer contact lenses. The commercial attitude results in extremes of price cutting so that deals can be made. Lenses may be given away at cost or even free if the deal can involve other purchases, payment for care and maintenance. Very often such offers are made to promote a new practice or new type of lens. In most cases the examination fees are extra, together with any special investigation. The high initial cost of fitting common in the UK may not in North America be more expensive than the 'give-away' deal offered via television and the newspapers.

Whatever the system, for anyone who can afford the initial outlay, the relative cost of lenses lessens in time. They need replacing as your sight alters, or if they are lost, when they should be replaced by insurance (see Chapter 5), while glasses are likely to need more frequent attention as both the frames and lenses are liable to be damaged.

In the next chapter we go into more detail about the types of contact lenses that are available, which are most suitable for the different eye conditions and how they are fitted. Your relationship with your specialist is very important from the beginning, and deciding whom to go to is the first decision to take. You will find advice on this too in Chapter 3.

3 CHOOSING AND FITTING CONTACT LENSES

Millions of people wear contact lenses. Perhaps your friend or colleague is wearing them right now without your realizing it. Some people keep their contact lenses a secret since they do not want anyone to know they have sight problems. But for most the ability to see well is a great victory over defective vision. Yet just because we have developed contact lenses so that many people are able to wear them successfully doesn't mean the story is finished. Every year better materials and methods of manufacture are invented and research is going on both at eye institutes and manufacturers' all over the world. You need to know what types are available and which would suit you best. This will ultimately be decided in discussion with your specialist. But it is useful to have some idea before you start.

What material are contact lenses made from?
The answer is simply plastic. But plastics are of several types, some hard like glass, others as soft as jelly. Some can absorb almost all their own weight in water, acting like transparent blotting paper. Generally, for contact lenses the softer the plastic the better the tolerance, since it is gentler on the eye, causing less pressure, and so is more comfortable. For some conditions, though, hard lenses are more effective (see pages 22, 87); and some people continue to wear them as they first started with contact lenses when only the harder plastics were available and prefer to continue with the type they are used to.

The first contact lenses were hard and dense – poor breathers – but now most are made of materials that breathe. In the same way sticky first-aid plasters (Band-aids) originally did not allow the passage of air and made the skin white and soggy, sometimes actually slowing down the healing of a wound.

What is the importance of lenses 'breathing'?
In Chapter 1 we saw how the eye is fed by the sticky tear fluid, and from the bloodstream, and by oxygen in the air reaching the exposed part of the eye through the tear film. With a contact lens covering the cornea, a lot of the external source of oxygen used to be lost. Glycogen in the cornea would be used up and the cornea would tend to swell, causing blurred vision. Although this is a temporary reaction it meant the lenses could be worn only for a few hours at a time.

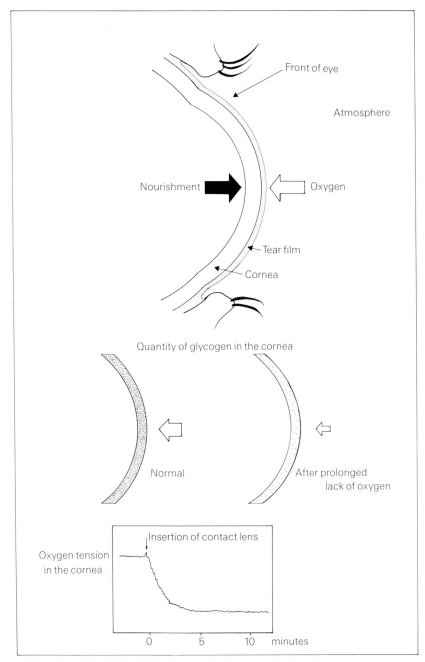

Front of eye

Atmosphere

Nourishment → ← Oxygen

Tear film

Cornea

Quantity of glycogen in the cornea

Normal

After prolonged
lack of oxygen

Insertion of contact lens

Oxygen tension
in the cornea

0   5   10   minutes

Above The eye is chiefly nourished from within and receives oxygen from the atmosphere; *centre*, glycogen is used up if there is an insufficient oxygen supply; *below*, a non-porous contact lens reduces this supply immediately it is inserted.

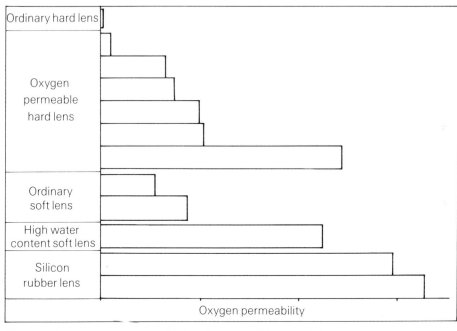

Ordinary hard lens			
Oxygen permeable hard lens			
Ordinary soft lens			
High water content soft lens			
Silicon rubber lens			

Oxygen permeability

Above   The oxygen permeability of different types of lenses.

Below   Corneal cells can be injured by contact lenses if the tear supply dries up.

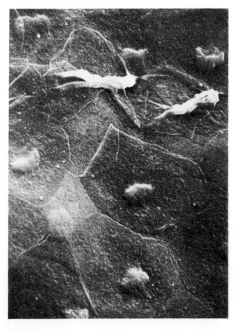

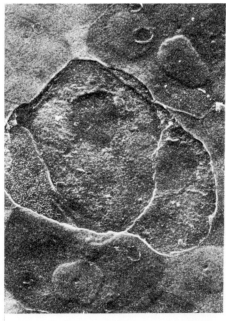

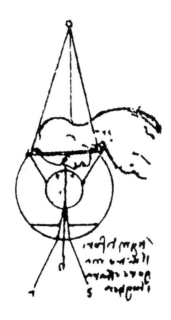

Leonardo da Vinci's drawing showing the principles of magnification through water.

The softer, porous lenses that began to be introduced during the mid-1970s have made it possible for wearers to keep their lenses in for days at a time, and sometimes even longer.

Developing the first contact lenses

You may have the impression that contact lenses have appeared in the last ten or twenty or thirty years; you would be wrong. The idea that vision could be corrected by looking through a glass bowl filled with water is almost five hundred years old, that is, a few years older than the first use of glasses in Europe. Leonardo da Vinci made some drawings showing that he understood the principles of magnification or reduction of images looked at through water. But it was not until the latter half of the nineteenth century that small semi-spherical glass bowls that fitted the eye were able to be blown from glass. They were first used to treat people with severe eye diseases and were sometimes filled with ointments. By the turn of the century these were being used to correct sight and there is evidence of German army officers wearing lenses in World War 1.

The first lenses, called scleral or haptic because they covered the

35

whole eyeball including the white, were filled with salt water of the same concentration as tears. Because they affected the eyes' breathing many people were unable to tolerate them, and even those who could suffered from sore red eyes after a few hours.

For many years the clinicians and contact lens fitters tried various ways of improving them. In the 1930s plastics began to be used and taking eye impressions became the practice. But discomfort continued to be a problem. Clinicians thought that the tear fluid under the contact lens was the chief difficulty and that after a short period of wear it became too acid. To counteract the acidity different alkaline solutions were tried, most of them containing bicarbonate. They did improve things a little. The most interesting fact that emerged was that a few people could tolerate a well-fitting large lens for several hours, although in the majority the sight became blurred after one to three hours. Even when holes were drilled in the lens to equalize the pressure between the front of the eye and the atmosphere and bring oxygen to the front of the eye, the wearing period was not increased for most people. Nevertheless, for the few who could tolerate them these large lenses were almost 100 per cent successful, producing no blurring of vision or discomfort. Why they have worked only for these people remains an unsolved puzzle. One possible explanation is that as the eyes move there is a pumping of tears from behind the lens to the outside.

How were smaller lenses developed?

An optician working in the United States called Tuohy fitted his wife with these plastic sclerals for near-sightedness and because she failed to adjust to them he made smaller and smaller versions until he designed a pair that she could tolerate. Thus was born the first corneal plastic contact lens, the forerunner of today's even smaller and thinner hard and semi-hard lenses.

The plastic used was an acrylate very similar to Perspex or Plexi-glass. At that time it was the softest material that was at the same time strong enough to be ground as a tiny lens. In the 1960s Otto Wychterle and Lim invented a new plastic that could absorb large quantities of water, making it softer and capable of containing the tear solution. This could at the same time be manufactured using a cheap means of production. It was the beginning of the soft plastic water contact lenses (hydrogels).

In the early days it was very difficult to get a plastics chemist from industry interested in the development of new plastics for contact lenses since the amounts required were so small. Today, with large corporations involved in contact lens manufacture, the story is very different. In fact the problem for wearers and specialists is that so many new materials appear on the market it is very difficult to assess their true value in comparison with those already in use.

There are plastics and plastics

An appropriate term to describe our present age would be the Plastic Age. We have had the Stone and the Iron Ages – and now the Plastic Age. Plastics are produced by making long sausage chains of one or more types of molecule that entwine themselves and then start to form a material. The plastic can be as hard as steel or as soft as butter. Before we knew the chemical secrets of plastics the human race was living with them – in fact from the beginning of history. Most living tissues and plant life are plastics. Substances such as rubber and resin are some of the raw materials from which we make refined plastic (silicon) contact lenses.

At present we have managed to develop durable materials that breathe but absorb very little or no water. We also have soft plastics that breathe and absorb a lot of water but are not so durable. In between there are rubber types that do not absorb water but breathe very nicely. Absorption is a very desirable quality because it softens the lens and makes it comfortable. It is also an additional way for oxygen to reach the eye. Many lenses that do not absorb water are given special coatings to make the eye tolerate them better and allow the mucous tear fluid to cover the surface easily.

What everyone is now trying to make is transparent hard and soft materials, able to breathe, cheap, that can be made into perfect lenses only a fraction of a millimetre in thickness, exactly reproduceable and yet strong enough to be handled by clumsy humans and in no way poisonous to human tissues. The research and trials to achieve this are endless. When a manufacturer invents a new lens it is extremely expensive to put on the market.

In future no doubt we shall be looking to more sophisticated combinations, with maybe hard-centred lenses that have soft surrounds, among others. The hard centre would be ideal for correcting such conditions as astigmatism, keratoconus and irregular corneas, while the softer surround would be comfortable and allow the eye to breathe.

What would be the ideal plastic from which to make a lens? First, it must be entirely transparent, then either by heat or injection moulding, or by some cutting procedure, able to be made into a very thin lens that once formed will not change its optical qualities even when handled by clumsy fingers. It must, when pressed between finger and thumb, as you put in the lens, be able to spring back to its original shape without snapping in two after a few times. The material should be durable enough not to degenerate over a short period, say, three years, not to absorb rays or other chemicals, even those of the body fluids, that would change its properties so that it would become spoilt by coatings. These are the most important qualities for an ideal lens plastic. There are many more dealing with such effects as the physical forces of electricity, how gases can pass through the material, and temperature. Thus if we ask for a material soft enough not to be felt, permeable enough not to interfere with the normal metabolism of the eye and yet work like a perfect optical lens you will see that the present situation is just a very good compromise and we hope in the future for even better plastics for contact lenses.

There are people who are highly motivated and want to try every new type that becomes available to find the best lenses. For many years Arthur was a successful contact lens wearer:

When he was sixteen years old – and this was in 1946 – Arthur read in the *Reader's Digest* that contact lenses of a new type were now being fitted. He persuaded his parents that it would be better for him if he could wear contact lenses. In fact, he was only a little near-sighted in each eye. Arthur was duly fitted and it took the best part of six months and several visits to an eye doctor and his technician to complete the task. The lenses were haptic, the large type that covered the whole of the front of the eye. They looked like miniature saucers when off the eye and measured a little more than 1 inch (2.5 cm) in diameter. Even this newest type could be worn by Arthur only for periods of six hours and then his eyes became red and his vision blurred. If he persisted longer than that his vision became so blurred that he could not even see with his glasses for several days. But he persevered and eventually could use the lenses for ten hours without too much blurring. On some occasions, especially if outdoors, Arthur could wear the lenses all day.

Ten years later, in 1955, he read about the new small lens and immediately went to a contact lens centre and was fitted. Needless to say, these were an unqualified success and he wore them all day and every day. Over the next five years Arthur went through a succession of fittings and lenses. Each pair of lenses was thinner and smaller than the last. And then in 1965 he read about the soft lenses and off he went and found the one practice in the city that had some, and he was fitted.

The following ten years saw Arthur trotting backwards and forwards to various contact lens specialists seeking newer types and even different colours. Arthur was hooked on contact lenses. Then a tragedy occurred. He developed a virus infection in his eyes and the result was an irritable sensation whenever the lenses were inserted so he was unable to tolerate any type, hard, soft or 'in between', large or small. But only a few months ago Arthur was still to be seen visiting doctors all over the world, hoping he could again become a successful

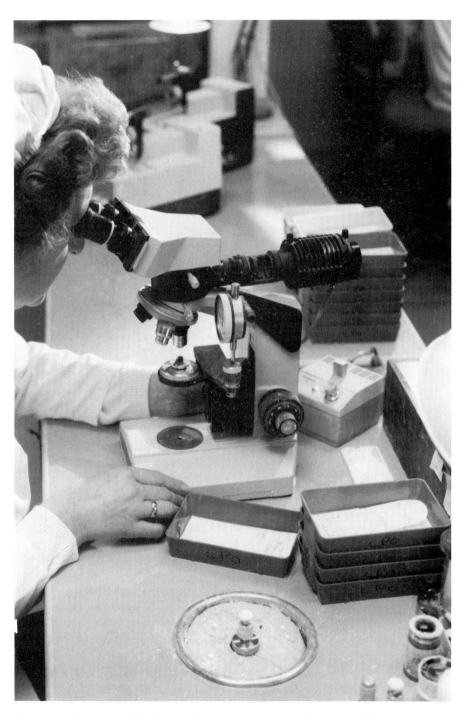

Final checking – verification of the base curves of a contact lens.

contact lens wearer. He said he would even have an operation to correct his eyesight if he could find someone to do it. Who knows – perhaps he has at last found someone!

The problem in Arthur's case was that his prolonged abuse of the eye tissue through overwear caused rejection of the lenses. If he hadn't forced such long periods of wear in the first place he might still be wearing lenses now.

How are contact lenses made?
The contact lens is a precision-made single item, manufactured, as we have said, since the early 1930s, from plastics. It was soon discovered that good lenses could be made either by cutting the lens shape with a lathe or by placing the fluid plastic into moulds. The plastic set in the mould and the machine coughed out thousands of lenses each day. Such a process often leads to a high rejection rate but nevertheless once the manufacturer has paid for the high cost of setting up the machine it is a cheap way of making lenses.

Whichever way the lenses were made, the advantages of speed and cheapness and the lightness of the lenses were soon recognized. Later, manufacturers became aware of the disadvantages of the lenses being too soft and spoiling easily during the cutting, and that badly made plastics changed colour and even lost their transparency. After half a century of development and research into plastics most of these problems have been solved. The more common manufacturing method is now by cutting the lens shape from large rods of plastic. The quality of the plastic varies according to the type of lenses being made – soft, semi-soft, rubbery or hard.

The fine processing for different degrees of far or near sight, or astigmatism, is done by hand. So many lenses are produced that there is every gradation of lens available, as there is with spectacle lenses.

The shape of the cornea
The surface of the cornea is, like a spectacle or camera lens, almost semi-spherical. It is very steeply curved at the centre just in front of the pupil and flatter towards the edge, nearer the white of the eye, and it does not have the same curvature from top to bottom as from side to side. For this reason we have to take care when we measure the curves so that a well-fitting lens is made – neither too steep nor too flat.

In the same way that we all have different sized heads, necks and so on, our corneal curves vary, so you would not expect to have exactly the same corneal curves as your spouse or best friend. People with big heads tend to have bigger eyes with flatter curves and women in general tend to have steeper curves than men because they have smaller eyes.

The fitting is a job for the contact lens specialist. To make sure that your lenses fit well, specialists now have instruments able to measure to the five-hundredth part of a millimetre the radius of curvature of the cornea. Not only that, but we have photographic equipment capable of recording the results of our measurements and even giving readings of other parts of the cornea that the edges of the contact lens will touch. For people with unusual curves contact lens fitting and correction of vision can be difficult and take quite a long time. Yet with the help of these fine instruments we can eventually produce lenses to suit just about everyone.

The way a lens is made, the material it is made from, the shape of the eye it will suit, whether it is good for daily wear or for several days at a stretch, are all factors that need consideration. There is no perfect contact lens material for everyone. Manufacturers may advertise contact lenses as they do motor cars and other products but in the final analysis it is the specialist, from his or her experience, expertise and knowledge about the availability of lenses, who will decide which is the

Hard lens sizes: now, a part of the cornea is exposed to the atmosphere (*left*), while previously a small hole was needed in the centre of the contact lens for oxygen (*right*).

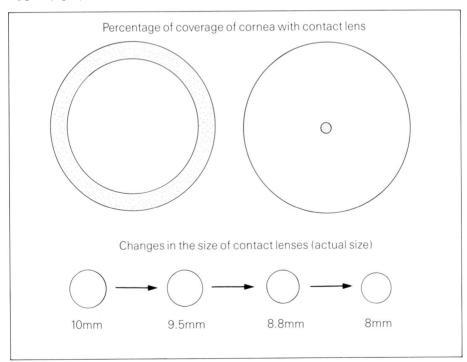

Percentage of coverage of cornea with contact lens

Changes in the size of contact lenses (actual size)

10mm   9.5mm   8.8mm   8mm

best for you. Your specialist will select the best lenses for tolerance and vision bearing all these points in mind:

- eye size and curvature
- lid movement
- hardness or softness of material
- gas permeability
- surface tolerance.

What size and thickness should your contact lens be?

The whole of the transparent cornea in front of the coloured part of the eye is about 12 to 13 mm in diameter. This is about the width of your middle fingernail. In fact, less than half of the area is used to form the picture that eventually arrives at the back of the eye, and that area is almost spherical. All contact lenses must be bigger than this central area to cover the field of vision effectively, so small hard lenses are rarely less than 8 mm in diameter, most are 9 to 10 mm and soft lenses between 12 and 15 mm in size. In general, large lenses do not move very much when you blink and they will give very good vision. One of the disadvantages of hard small lenses is that they can move a lot over the eye as it moves or the lids blink, and if they are too small your sight can come and go.

The thickness of lenses varies according to lens power and material. For some (minus or minifying power) lenses, centre thicknesses as little as 0.03 mm are possible. But the ideal thickness has to be based on factors such as optical quality and how much oxygen can pass through the material.

Plus lenses (magnifying) have their greatest thickness at the centre and therefore the lens design uses the smallest area for the power of lens as possible to correct the sight. The rest of the contact lens is as thin as possible. So it is misleading for manufacturers to advertise, as they sometimes do, one lens as better than another because of its gas permeability. It is the lens design and thickness for the power needed by the wearer that decide this property.

The table opposite is no more than a rough guide to the many types of contact lens available. Obviously lenses can be made of either hard or soft materials, to all powers and thicknesses – and even all colours. Why are there so many variables and how do you know which is the best lens for you?

Since all contact lenses are an extra burden on the eye, the thinnest and smallest that give good vision must be the ideal. Apply this to the different materials, hard and soft, and the wearer's needs, and you can

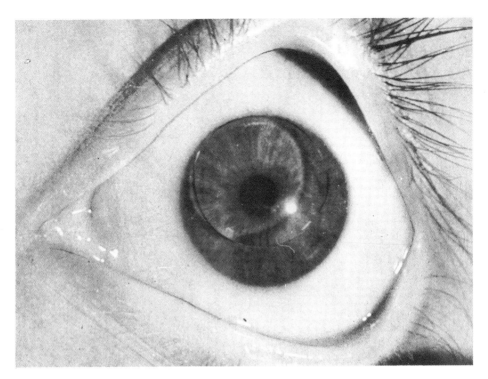

A hard corneal lens that has moved off the centre of the eye.

Lens type	Size
Corneal (hard)	
Mini	7.5–8.5 mm
Intermediate	8.5–11 mm
Scleral (soft)	
Mini	12–13 mm
Intermediate	13–15 mm
Haptic (large hard or soft scleral)	15–24 mm

Extended wear
Any lens that allows sufficient ventilation of oxygen to the cornea while the wearer is asleep can be used for extended wear.

Common types of lenses.

Qualities	Hard gas permeable	Soft rubber	Soft water gel
Sucks on to eye	a little	often	sometimes
Feels hard	always	sometimes	seldom
Adaptation time	3–12 weeks	1–3 weeks	1 day–3 weeks depending on whether worn daily or extended wear
Maintainence	easy	frequent cleaning and disinfection	frequent cleaning and disinfection
Wetting of lens and comfort	variable	poor to fair	good
Durability	several years	1–2 years	6 months–2 years

Qualities of common types of contact lens.

see why some contact lenses have to be larger and others thicker than might seem necessary at first.

A small, thin lens must centre on the eye to function, and unless it can adhere to the eye it will fall off every time the eyes blink or move suddenly. Therefore the softer the material the larger the lens has to be.

To correct sight successfully the back of the lens needs to imitate the shape of the individual eyeball, whereas the front is made to the normal eyeball shape. So for some people, a very thin lens cannot be fitted. On the other hand, a thicker lens will sometimes produce suction on the front of the eye, which is damaging to the eye tissue.

The aim in fitting is always to allow sufficient movement over the eye surface for the normal blinking of the lids. Yet the movement must not be excessive or it would cause erratic vision and could not be tolerated.

Gas permeability
How does the eye breathe if it is covered with a contact lens? There are two possibilities:

1. The front of the eye can obtain oxygen through the lens material and pass back waste gases in the opposite direction;

2. The tears around and under the lens can carry the gases. In this case the contact lens must fit loosely enough to allow the tears to flow.

Both hard and soft lenses follow these principles of breathing and pumping fluids, although soft lenses have very little pumping action.

Larger lenses are popular and now even the large scleral (haptic) lenses still worn by a few people (see page 36) are made successfully from gas permeable materials. These people therefore at last have a more comfortable lens that can be worn for several hours each day.

How long can different types be worn?

This is a rather complicated question to answer. It depends not only on your own tolerance but also on the material of the lens and the fitting as to:

1. How much oxygen can reach the eye over a certain time;

2. How easily all the microscopic waste products that accumulate on the eye surface can be cleared without causing problems.

As we explained above, the newer plastics are mostly gas permeable, so newly fitted lenses usually allow more oxygen to reach the eye than the older, hard lenses. The softer the lens the more gas permeable it is. The very large soft (scleral) lenses cover a bigger area, obviously preventing oxygen reaching more of the eye than small lenses. So despite their high permeability they may not allow more oxygen to a particular wearer's eye than the harder type.

Size also affects keeping the lens clean in the eye. Your tears have to wash and wipe the lens in the same way as they normally wash and wipe the eyeball (see Chapter 1). But as the lens is an extra thickness and made of different material, the tears have to work harder and both the size and type of the lenses will affect the way your tears work.

Some lenses can be worn only during the day, while others can also be slept in. But the time you can keep your lenses in is not as important as good vision and tolerance.

So it will be a matter of luck whether yours can remain in your eyes for a long time or not. The table on page 46 is a guide to the periods different types can normally be worn.

Lens type	Average daily wear	Extended wear
Hard materials		
Non-breathing corneal	8–15 hours	—
Breathing corneal (gas permeable)	10–18 hours	5–7 days (special types only)
Scleral	4–10 hours	—
Gel soft materials		
Ultra-thin low water content	12–16 hours	7–14 days
Normal thickness gel	8–16 hours	—
High water content	12–16 hours	7–14 days
Silica gel (rubber) soft	8–16 hours	2–5 days

Rest periods vary according to advice from the specialist. One in 7 days is common for all except silicon soft, when 1 in 5 is usually recommended.

Wearing time for different types of lenses.

Extended wear lenses
These can be of either hard or soft materials. They must be guaranteed by the manufacturer as suitable for extended wear – not all powers are possible in the extended wear materials. The success rate for young people is about 80 per cent for soft and 70 per cent for hard. Wearers are usually advised to remove the lenses once a week for cleaning and a night's rest (see also page 65) and soft extended wear lenses should be renewed every six months, making them expensive. The chances of infection are at present greater than with daily wear. Using the wrong materials, bad fitting of the lenses or bad follow-up treatment can lead to serious problems in extended wear.

Choosing a specialist
Deciding whom to go to for your contact lenses may be straightforward – perhaps a relative or friend who already has lenses can recommend a first-class optometrist. If you don't know of anyone, you may not want to take chances by going to the first person you hear about. The qualifications for contact lens fitters vary widely from country to country.

In the UK opticians, optometrists and ophthalmologists (eye specialists) can fit lenses. (A dispensing optician must work to a prescription from an ophthalmologist or optometrist.) In Japan only medical eye specialists are allowed to fit lenses. In North America an ophthalmologist usually tests your eyes and provides a prescription, and an optician fits the lenses. In any event, an optometrist or eye doctor should provide the prescription even if the lenses are fitted by a non-specialist, but this is not always observed; and in some countries there are no regulations whatsoever, so a jeweller or drug store technician can fit the lenses.

Obviously, we recommend you go to someone who is qualified, whether an ophthalmologist or an optometrist or optician. You may pay more, but prescribing the right lenses and getting the best fit will mean the difference between long-term success and failure. Of course there are people who succeed with a quickly fitted pair bought from a highly commercialized outlet, but the chances are lower and it is hardly worth the risk when you're taking such an important step. Although fitting most wearers is becoming easier, the aftercare is developing into a speciality. This is the most expensive part of contact lens maintenance and determines the overall success for many people. It requires the greatest expertise when problems arise.

Select a few names showing the proper qualification and have a look at their premises. A clean, well-run clinic with up-to-date equipment is a good indication of an efficient practice. Ask the cost of prescribing and fitting. You can find out the average price in your area by getting several quotes (though the specialist can give only a very rough idea before he or she knows exactly which lenses you need). As with any job, don't necessarily go for the cheapest.

Your relationship with your specialist
Any relationship takes time to build, and as with your doctor or dentist, once you have got to know each other and have worked through problems together, you will have built up a valuable store of information. It is worth keeping the same specialist, if possible, even if you move to another district.

Having your eyes tested
Whether you have your eyes examined at an ophthalmologist's or at an optometrist's, the tests for focusing will be basically the same.

Distance vision You will be asked to read a chart with letters of decreasing size at a distance of 20 feet (6 metres). If you are able to read the chart almost to the bottom you will have normal vision, known as 6/6 in the UK, 20/20 in North America. If you can read only the top line your vision is recorded as 6/60, or 20/200.

Near vision You are given a piece of print with different-sized type on it and asked to read it at your normal reading distance. (You have to remember that working distances can be different from reading distances.)

From these tests the specialist will find out whether you have near or far sight, or astigmatism. It can then be decided whether your eyes are suitable for contact lenses, or whether glasses would be better (see Chapter 1).

4 WHO WEARS CONTACT LENSES?

The proportion of people wearing glasses varies in different countries. A lot depends on racial characteristics. Some races seem more likely to develop near sight (see Chapter 2), in others cataract is more common, so there is sometimes a need for glasses or contact lenses after operation. If one had to put a round figure on the number of people who need glasses, it would at present be 15 per cent of people up to the age of thirty, and over forty pretty well everyone (for reading). The need for sight correction for the whole world goes into many millions of people. A proportion of the people who need glasses wear contact lenses. In the UK, possibly 2 to 3 million wear contact lenses and in the USA the figure is put at 20 million or about one-twelfth of the population.

When are they most useful?

Occupation

- Since they are so successful for distance vision (see Chapter 1) contact lenses are especially useful for near-sighted people leading active lives, for example, sportsmen and dancers and people in the armed forces on active service.

- For water sports contact lenses can be worn under swimming goggles. For sports such as water polo and even boxing large scleral lenses are suitable.

- Since they do not steam over in the hot and humid atmospheres of kitchens or, at the other extreme, in a cold atmosphere, as in a cold storage room, lenses are also very useful for people in catering and the food industry.

- People in heavy industry who need to wear goggles, for example, steel workers, can wear contact lenses successfully. The goggles fit better without glasses and at the same time the eyes are protected by both lenses and goggles. The lenses do not, though, protect the eyes from dangerous ultra-violet or infra-red light, unless they are made from a special filtering material.

- Contact lenses are invaluable when appearance is important – for actors and photographic models, or public figures such as politicians, as well as just for people who prefer their looks without glasses.

Are there any occupations where they are unsuitable?
- In jobs where there is a lot of close work such as constant reading, or working with fine instruments or jewellery – and especially if lighting is poor – contact lenses will not give the best long-term results (as explained in Chapter 2, they are better for distance vision). Nevertheless, for people who see better with them than glasses, even in these occupations they will on balance be preferable.

- Excessive air pollution, dry air or flash welding are examples of atmospheres in the workplace that would make contact lenses unwearable.

Different ages

Babies
Babies can be given contact lenses at any age. The reasons your baby may need to wear lenses would be for a serious optical defect such as extreme near sight, or high astigmatism or strabismus (see Chapter 2); the lenses will develop better sight, where glasses would be impractical. It would be extremely difficult, if not impossible, to have a young baby wear glasses continuously. When a congenital cataract has been removed, a contact lens is inserted. This, though, is a very rare condition in babies (see Chapter 8 for more on cataracts).

Your baby has to be assessed for his or her suitability with regard to:

1. Type of lens

2. Wearing time

3. Personality.

If the results show lenses to be a positive advantage, the baby will be measured and fitted in the same way as an adult. The lenses prescribed are nearly always daily wear rather than extended wear. These are safest as daily checking and cleaning reduce the chances of infections developing. Extended wear lenses are used rarely. If it is decided they are preferable, you have to be well trained by your practitioner on how to check your baby's eyes frequently and periodically to clean the lenses thoroughly (more detailed advice on putting in lenses and cleaning is given in Chapter 5).

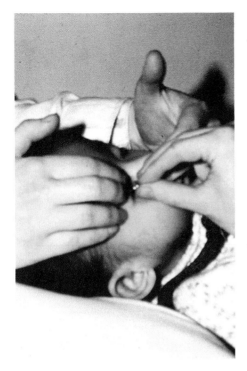

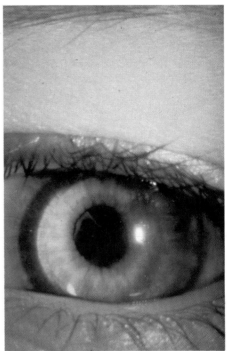

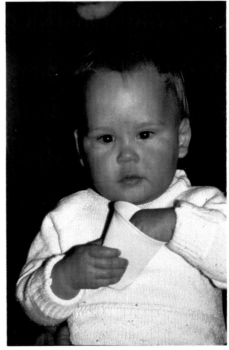

A baby with congenital cataract who was first fitted with contact lenses at twelve weeks. By the age of two, he was able to see normally (*bottom right*).

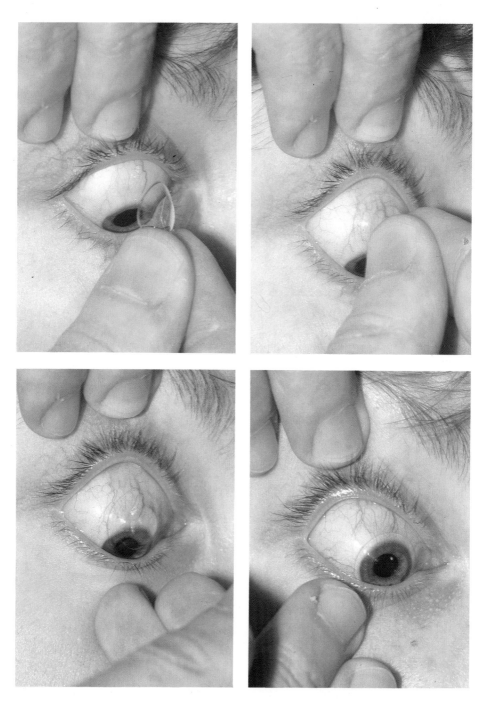

Inserting contact lenses into an elderly person's eyes, whose fingers are not mobile enough for the job.

Children

For children lenses are usually better than glasses, not only because they avoid the possibility of accidents from broken glass or frames, but also because children don't like the discomfort of glasses and usually prefer not to have their looks altered. Glasses can make them self-conscious and that may mean they stop wearing them when they think they can get away with it. If the sight defect is strabismus, constant wear is important (see Chapter 2), so contact lenses are a better solution. Wearing contact lenses may even cure painful shyness, as in Emma's case:

Emma was twelve years old when it was decided that her near sight was bad enough to wear glasses all the time. She was a quiet girl. She stayed at home, rarely went out and about like her schoolmates. She read books at home; watched television; did her mother's hair and her sister's. She could run the 100 metres in 17.7 seconds but tried hard to keep her name off any list for sports events or team games. Her shyness was a worry to her parents. Her dislike of glasses became an obsession. She would often purposely forget to bring them home from school and then screw up her eyes trying to see. Neighbours thought Emma peculiar. She never returned a smile or a nod of recognition.

Emma's mother one day had to collect her from school and take her shopping. Emma was now fourteen and fast developing into a young woman. While waiting, her mother got into conversation with a few other mothers and was told about one girl in Emma's class who wore contact lenses and had become literally a new person.

Emma's mother thought they should give lenses a try. Emma was successfully fitted and she changed within three months into an outward going personality. She dressed differently, did her hair with style and had a hoard of friends. It was even rumoured that she was on the way to becoming a class prefect, and would one day be in the running for school captain.

Elderly people

There is no upper age limit for wearing contact lenses. But they sometimes have to be abandoned when the wearer's fingers become arthritic so that putting the lenses in and removing them is difficult. Then there is a danger of infections starting up, or even injury if the lens has become uncomfortable and cannot be removed.

There is also the problem of confusion and forgetfulness in some older people. Caring for your lenses is very important (see Chapter 5) and when personal daily hygiene is no longer easy, contact lenses should not be worn.

Yet contact lenses are often prescribed after cataract operations, more common in the elderly than any other age group (see Chapter 8). When either the problems of mobility or forgetfulness occur after a cataract operation it is essential that someone in the household becomes responsible for the care, insertion and removal of the lens.

Dry eyes are more common in older people too (see Chapter 1), and they of course make wearing contact lenses difficult. If the condition can't be put right with suitable eye drops it may be necessary to wear glasses instead.

5 GETTING TO KNOW YOUR LENSES

In the first four chapters we have talked a lot about the theory of lenses. Now we shall deal with the practical aspects of wearing them. Even successful wearers fall into bad habits with their lenses, usually with minor consequences. In this book we want to make both prospective and habitual contact lens wearers aware of all the problems and how to avoid them.

Putting your lenses in

The first exercise to learn is putting the lenses in and out of the eye. From birth we are taught that the eyes are sensitive and not to be touched, and to avoid anything likely to hit the eye. We instinctively protect our eyes by closing the lids or putting our hands up to ward off flying objects. Suddenly you are asked deliberately to put something in the eye. Most people find that by reflex they close both eyes and keep them closed. It takes a little time to get used to keeping both eyes open. They water, both from lack of blinking and in reaction to the lenses. But eventually the tear reflex stops and putting in contact lenses becomes a habit.

You will be shown how to put in and take out your lenses by your specialist. However, the following steps are a useful guide and reminder when you are getting into practice at home. As you become more used to the procedure you will be able to cut out a lot of the steps and put the lenses in very quickly. To begin with it is best to follow the guidelines closely. That way you will both get into the good habit of keeping the lenses scrupulously clean, and you will avoid any unnecessary discomfort.

1. Sit at a clean table top with a mirror at eye level. Place the lens container in front of you, together with a clean, non-fluffy tissue, which you can use to dry any excess tears. Make sure your hands are clean.

2. Remove one lens from the container. Make sure it is clean, ready for putting in the eye. It is sometimes advisable to rinse the lens if the storage solution has a strong chemical in it; the directions on

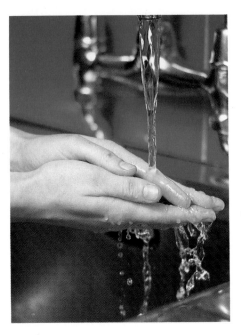
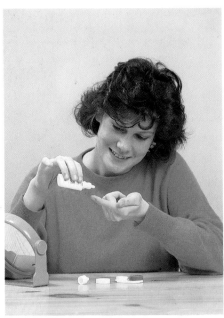

Inserting lenses: 1. Wash your hands. 2. Rinse your lens, if directed. 3. Place the clean lens on your index finger.

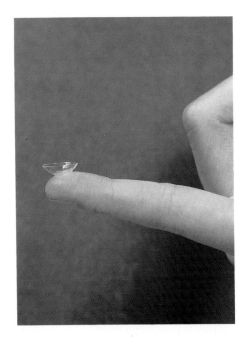

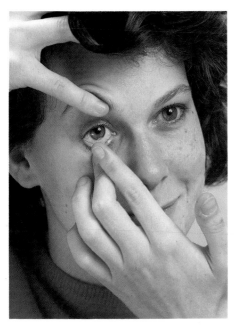
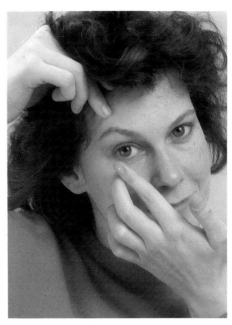

4. Soft lens: hold the upper lid open with the other hand and insert the lens.
5. Hard lens: the technique is the same, but try to position the lens on the centre of the eye. 6. If necessary, a hard lens can be centred by gently massaging your eyelid.

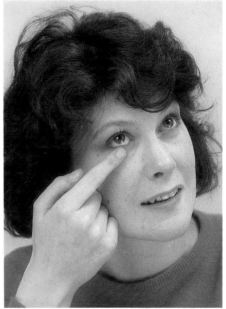

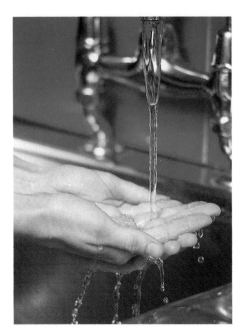
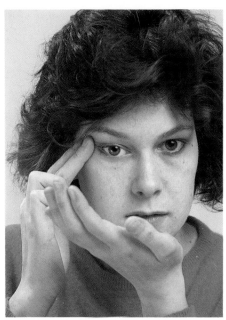

Removing lenses: 1. Wash your hands first. 2. Hard lenses: cup your lower hand to receive the lens. 3. A rubber sucker may be used to remove a hard lens.

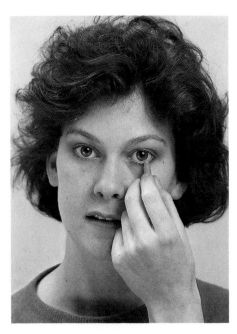

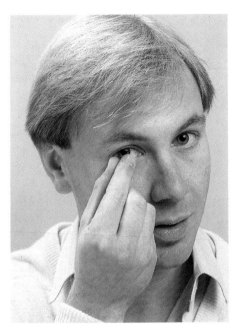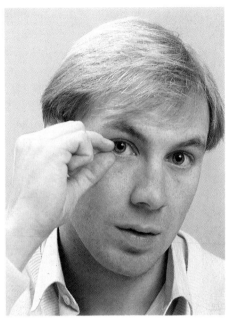

4. Soft lenses: pinch below the centre of the lens to remove. 5. Rubber lenses: pinch off from the side of the eye. 6. Clean your lenses and store them in the proper solution.

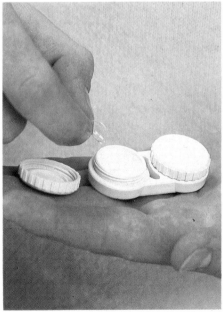

the bottle will tell you what to do (see also page 65). *Do not* wet the lens in your mouth: your spit may contain germs.

3. Place the clean lens on the index finger of the hand you write with. The lens should now look like a little bowl with the inside uppermost. If the lens is very soft and floppy, let it dry for a minute or two while on your finger and it will form a more rigid shape.

4. With the other hand, hold the upper lid open. While looking with both eyes into the mirror with your head lowered, place the lens on the coloured part (iris) of the eye.

5. Repeat with the second lens.

A soft lens will gradually centre itself. A hard lens will not, and if not positioned right at first it may go under the lid – but it cannot go behind the eye as some people think (see the eye's anatomy in Chapter 1 and you will realize it can't go beyond the lid). Wherever the hard lens goes, it can be massaged and directed on to the pupil area. You should close your eye and gently apply pressure to your eyelid.

Removing your lenses

The technique for doing this is according to the type of lens you wear (see the photographs on pages 58–9).

1. Again, remember to wash your hands first.

2. **Hard lenses:** pressure and tightening the lids will flick out the lenses, so make sure your hand is cupped to receive them. A rubber sucker may be used.

3. **Soft lenses:** pinch below the centre of the lens, with a backward squeeze, between the lids.

4. **Rubber lenses:** push the lens to the white of the eye with the index finger and pinch off slowly below the centre with finger and thumb.

5. Whenever lenses are removed they should be cleaned immediately. Keep them in their container in their proper storage solution (see page 65). Rinse as recommended before reinserting them into your eyes.

What should you do if you cannot remove your contact lenses?
Don't panic. If the conventional methods fail, do not apply pressure to the eye. If you are wearing hard lenses and they are on the cornea, place

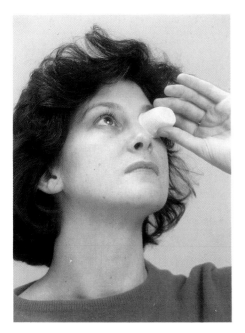
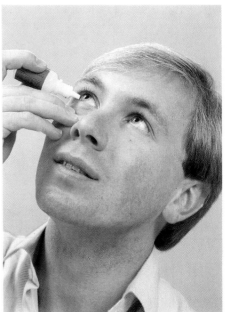
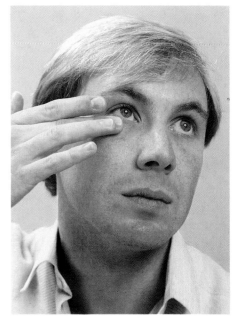

If you cannot remove a lens: 1. Hard corneal lenses – place an eye bath over your eye and blink. 2. For soft lenses – put saline drops, supplied by your practitioner, in your eye. 3. Pinch the edge of the lens.

your eye open in a bowl of water or eye bath and blink. If you are wearing soft lenses use saline eyedrops (artificial tears). These can be obtained from your practitioner and you should always keep some available. Put the drops in your eyes and gently pinch the edge of the lens to break the suction.

How long will it take to learn to put in your lenses? The first time you will need help from your practitioner. Most people master the principles of putting in and taking out their lenses at their first session in about an hour. Getting practised enough to put them in with one finger without holding open the lids or needing a mirror will probably take a few weeks. But once you have reached this stage, it is easy to fall into bad habits, forgetting or not worrying about using clean hands and keeping the lenses rinsed. This can lead to infections and spoiling your lenses so it is important to follow the advice in this chapter.

Getting used to your lenses

How long will it take for your lenses to become so comfortable you can even forget you are wearing them? From the beginning will power and determination are essential. Long-term success depends on the sensitivity of the wearer and the environment, and it also varies with the different types of lens.

Hard lenses
These are certainly more difficult to adjust to because of the material. The edges of the lenses can be felt against the eyelids and to begin with may make your eyes sore. The reaction is for your eyelids to drag against the extra thickness so you want to blink repeatedly or keep your eyes half closed. You will also find your eyes water a lot for the first few days.

As long as your lenses have been fitted well, your eyes are moist enough and you don't develop any irritating condition, you should get used to hard lenses in three to four weeks. Successful hard lens wearers can then keep them in all day, however late they stay up at night. It does take perseverance, though, and a lot of wearers (about 30 per cent) find they cannot get on with hard lenses because of the uncomfortable lens-to-lid sensation. A softer type may be comfortable and if they give good vision your specialist will try them as an alternative.

Soft lenses
It is often possible for daily wearers to keep them in for several hours, even on the first day, and about 80 per cent will adapt within one week. The thinner, softer material makes them far less uncomfortable on the eye than the hard lenses.

62

Extended or constant wear lenses

These are frequently kept in for several days or even weeks from the time they are first fitted; again, one week is the average time it takes to get used to the sensation of a foreign body in the eye.

Extended wear lenses are not suitable for everyone, although their convenience makes them the most attractive. Even after succeeding with them at the beginning your eyes can become intolerant so that you have to go back to another type:

Julie had been long-sighted since infancy – in fact, at one time the child clinic thought she had a squint and exercises had been advised. However, the eye that tended to turn in when she was tired had reasonably good vision. Between the ages of four and eleven she had to wear glasses all the time but since she could see just as well without them they stayed in her school bag or locker more often than on her nose.

At college she found that she had to use them to get through the large amount of reading there was to do. At parties, after a few drinks, she was alarmed to see herself in a mirror with a terrible turning in of the eye. At a party a giggling girl with a cross-eye is definitely not attractive. So Julie went to see her optician and was advised to wear glasses all the time. They certainly kept her eyes straight but she did not like herself with glasses – neither the small round gold frames trying to look like a Victorian girl nor the ravishing upswept Batman wings that made her feel like someone at the Mardi Gras. The obvious alternative was contact lenses.

Unfortunately Julie had sensitive skin, with some eczema. When the optician tried to test her with small hard corneal lenses she passed out completely for several seconds. Nevertheless, she persevered and tried soft lenses. She was very successful wearing them up to twelve hours each day, and continued to be able to for eight years.

Last summer she went to New York and saw on the television there advertisements for lenses you can sleep in and don't need removing for up to thirty days. Julie made an appointment to see her optician after she returned home. He said these lenses were available, but frequently required taking out in under thirty days. More than one new pair a year was often necessary. But Julie went ahead and for three months had the thrill of waking up in the morning and being able to see well without the bother of putting in contact lenses.

Suddenly, on waking after a party where everyone had been smoking, she had sticky lids, red eyes, blurred vision and a discharge from the eyes. She tried to take out the lenses but panicked when she found it difficult and rushed off to the hospital. Her eyes had an infection and the lenses were removed. Julie was treated with eyedrops and after a week was better. She tried to wear her lenses again but could not. Immediately after putting them in, her eyes became red and watery and even painful. This went on for several weeks and in despair, even after seeing a specialist, she had to return to wearing glasses.

It was not until two years later that Julie's eyes could tolerate lenses again, and this time she went back to daily wear soft lenses and had to be very careful to avoid all irritating chemicals that some contact lens solutions contain.

Julie's story points again to how important follow-up visits and aftercare are for successful long-term wear.

Follow-up visits

For daily wear lenses   After the first visit, you will probably need to see the specialist at least once more to make sure the lenses fit well and are comfortable. This can be properly assessed only after you have had a chance to get used to them. Once you and the specialist are satisfied your lenses are right for vision and comfort you will need to go back from time to time to have your eyes tested for changes in your sight. Your specialist will tell you how often you will need to make these visits.

For extended wear lenses   The specialist will need to check how you are adapting to extended wear lenses after the first twenty-four hours, or certainly within the first week, and you will probably need to make several further follow-up visits; after one month and again after three and six months.

If you have any discomfort with your lenses that you can't put right yourself you will have to get advice. We go into more detail about this when we discuss looking after your lenses in this chapter, and in Chapter 6.

Looking after your lenses

There are snags to every lens and material because nature never intended a piece of plastic to be worn over the eye. For example, if wet (soft) lenses are not stored correctly when they are not being worn they can become infected and spoilt. Any lens treated roughly can scratch or tear. And desposits from eye discharges or from chemicals in the storage solution can spoil the surface. Modern contact lenses are made from soft and easily spoiled plastics. Since they are expensive it is important to know how to keep them as long as possible.

Storing your lenses
Both hard and soft lenses must be stored in solution. The storage solution provided with your new lenses will be the correct type for them, and you should use only that type in your lens container. It would be pointless to list all the preparations currently available in the world (nearly 200) since many are the same but with different names, and every month a new one is announced and another may be discontinued. The advice of both your specialist and the manufacturer is essential. Solvents carelessly or wrongly used can result in an inflamed eye.

The solution in your contact lens container must be emptied and refilled with fresh fluid every twenty-four hours when in use, otherwise the solution and lens can become spoilt and infected. Most solutions have two dates that must be remembered. One is the length of time the solution will remain usable while the bottle is unopened, the other how long it can be used after it is opened. Once a bottle has been opened the contents can become infected. So it is important to use the solution within the stated time and then throw away the bottle. Never top up an old bottle with solution to use at work, as it can harbour germs.

Cleaning your lenses
Hard lenses should always be rinsed in clean water before insertion and after removal unless a special wetting solution has been advised. Soft lenses may be cleaned before storage with a special solution, or with a solvent added to the storage solution. These are provided by the manufacturer. As long as you store the lenses in their solution, and follow the manufacturer's instructions on rinsing – if needed – before insertion, they should always be clean and ready to wear.

Extended wear lenses need cleaning with their recommended solvent at regular intervals – about once a week – to remove greasy or sticky particles; again, follow the manufacturer's instructions carefully. If the lenses are not going to be reinserted for several hours, a disinfectant solution must be used.

All lenses that have to be stored in the wet state also need occasional sterilization to kill any germs that may be present on the lens or in the storage solution. The methods are either by heating the special chemical solution provided for this purpose in an electrical heater or saucepan of water and putting in the lens in their container, or by placing them in the cold solution for several hours.

Sometimes these sterilizing solutions have to be rinsed off or a neutralizer used before you can put the lens back in the eye. You should always read the instructions on the label very carefully and if in doubt

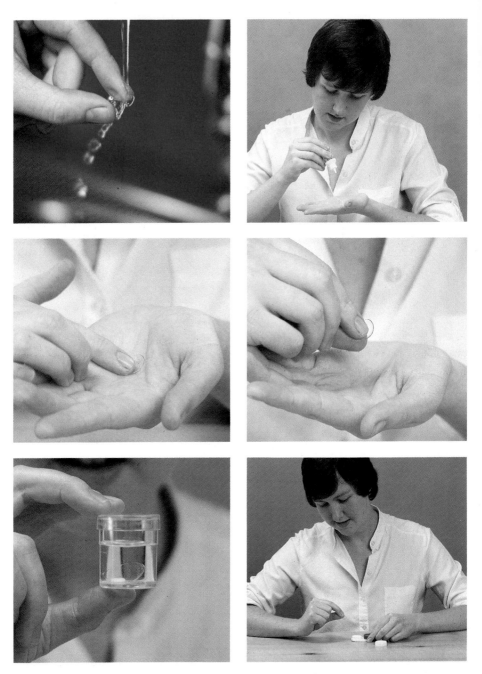

1. Clean hard lenses by rinsing in clean water. 2. Soft lenses: put drops of the cleaning solution in the palm of your hand. 3. Cleaning with a circular motion. 4. Rubbing between finger and thumb. 5. Periodically soak soft lenses in a protein removing solution. 6. Always store your lenses in their proper solution.

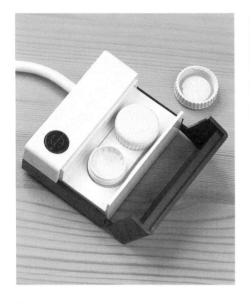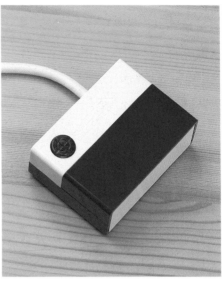

Sterilizing soft lenses in an electrical heater: *left*, the lenses are placed in saline solution. *Right* The machine is closed for the specified cycle – 25–45 minutes.

ask the specialist or technician who supplied the lenses which method to use and exactly how to follow it.

Spoiling of a lens

Deposits of mucous, grease, cosmetics and débris from the eye or the hands may together with water cause fungus to grow on a badly maintained soft lens. If protein from the tears changes and dries on the lens it can make the surface uncomfortable and rough. It may even become unwettable. All these effects are usually avoided by keeping your lenses clean with the correct cleaning solution. But you may be given a protein or lipid remover as an additional cleaning solution if your lenses often become coated with eye secretions. This must be rinsed off before you put your lenses in or you will have hazy vision.

If your lenses become so heavily ingrained that you can't clean them, you should take them to the specialist, who will try stronger cleaning solutions. If these don't work, the lenses may be sent to the manufacturer, who can use machine methods. But the cleaning process itself can spoil the surface so that even though a lens looks clean it may be rough and uncomfortable to wear. A new lens is better than a chemically cleaned dirty one. Changing soft lenses several times a year would be ideal but too expensive at present.

What happens when lenses age?

1. The plastic will deteriorate and this can give a yellow-brown tinge

2. Or it can go cloudy

3. Soft lenses lose their suppleness and take on an abnormal appearance

4. The edges may become rough or cracked

5. Hard lenses can craze over the surface

6. Deposits of all colours can appear on the surface.

Left The surface of a soft contact lens spoilt by protein; *right*, a soft contact lens surface (magnified) showing mould.

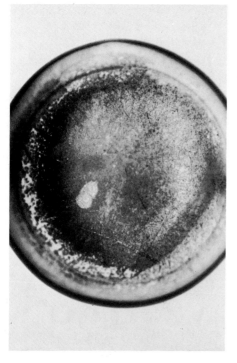 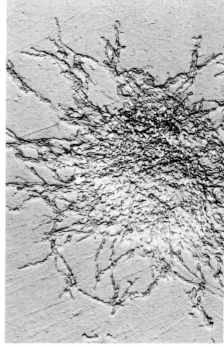

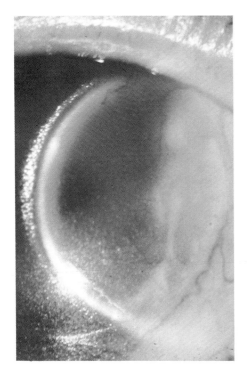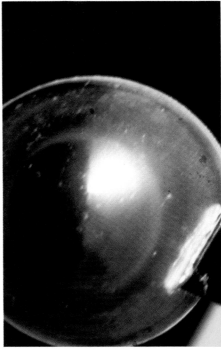

Examples of contact lenses that have been spoilt by discoloration or crazing.

If you are getting bad or blurred vision, you will obviously need a new pair of lenses. Wearing scratched or discoloured lenses will not make your sight worse, but it will make seeing a lot more difficult. The time you will be able to keep your lenses depends on your own maintenance, as we have said, and on the material. The table on page 44 gives a very rough guide to the life of the different types.

Losing lenses

This is one of the main worries for contact lens wearers. A lens can, occasionally, fall out, say if there is a strong blast of wind that hits the eye at an angle and lifts the lens off, or if by mistake you open your eyes under water. When you are not wearing your lenses, it is easy to mishandle these tiny objects as you try to put them in. You may drop them and then have to try and find them when your sight is poor. How can you avoid this annoying problem?

1. Don't put them on in an unsuitable place such as a bus or a train.

2. Don't be in a hurry.

3. If your sight is very poor *do* wear a pair of glasses until you're ready to insert the lenses.

4. Make sure the room is well lit so that if you drop a lens you have the best chance of finding it.

5. Always keep a spare case for your lenses at work as well as at home so that when you take them out you can store them safely.

Insurance

You should anyway be prepared for loss or damage by insuring your lenses as soon as you buy them. This can be done in several ways and your specialist will advise you. Here are some options:

1. Insurance for loss and theft can be included in your own household or travel policy.

2. There is special contact lens insurance to cover accidental breakage and loss during wear available from major insurance companies.

3. Replacement maintenance schemes at low cost are offered by many specialists. These may also include the specialist's fees for after care. For example:

Cost of lenses plus fitting lenses $= x$
1 year's maintenance plus percentage of replacement $= y$
Total cost for first year $= x + y$

These practical points of fitting and maintenance will be important to you from the moment you start wearing contact lenses. In the next chapter we go into more detail about problems that can arise later, when you are a habitual wearer.

6 ADAPTING TO YOUR LENSES

In the last chapter we explained how it takes time and perseverance to get used to wearing lenses. Looking after your lenses and keeping them clean ensures comfortable wear. Yet there will be later problems, however well fitted they are, and even for the people who usually tolerate their lenses well. This chapter shows what those problems are and how they can be overcome.

Common causes of discomfort

The human eye is well supplied by nerves since it is a delicate organ that must be protected against injury. These nerves are particularly sensitive to small irregular foreign bodies like dust particles. Im-

Two conditions that can affect contact lens wearers: blepharitis, *left*, and conjunctivitis, *right*.

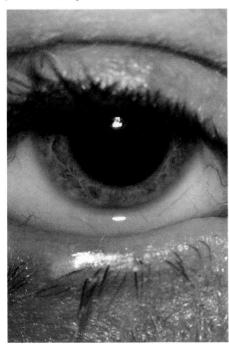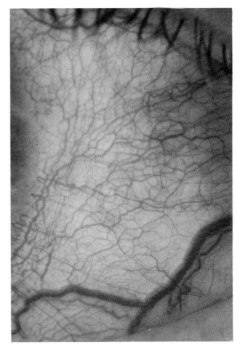

mediately they are irritated the eye produces tears as a reflex action and the lids either blink or remain closed, whichever is the more successful in stopping the painful sensation and removing the irritants.

If you feel sudden discomfort This can be due to the lens moving in your eye, because of grit or a dust particle getting into your eye and even behind the lens. Sudden drying up of the tears can cause pain too.

You should remove the lens, let your eyes water, wash it with clear water or its special solvent, which is then rinsed off, and replace it. But make sure you wait until your eye is comfortable before putting the lens in again or you will irritate the soreness.

Irritant fumes will cause the same reflex reactions as grit or dust. Some are found only at work. If your job involves working with chemicals likely to irritate your eyes you should be given protective goggles. But other chemicals giving off fumes are used in the home, such as chlorine from bleach, turpentine, alcohol, glues and paint solvents. Vapours from aerosols such as hair sprays, deodorizers and insect repellants can be accidentally directed into the eye. They dissolve into the tear film and irritate the eye tissue. Obviously you should avoid them whenever you can; but if you do get fumes that make your eyes smart, you should take out your lenses and not put them back until the soreness has completely disappeared.

Wearing your lenses too long, if they are for limited-period wear, will make your eyes sore. Your specialist will advise you during the first visit how long you should keep the lenses in. Don't exceed the time because of, say, an unexpected social engagement. Carry a pair of glasses with you and change to them when your lenses have been in the maximum time.

At first you will probably not want to keep the lenses in the full time anyway. The ability to wear contact lenses increases with practice and you shouldn't be discouraged because you can wear them only for short periods during the first few weeks (see also Chapter 5).

Dry, smoky atmospheres Smoke will irritate your eyes in the same way as other fumes. It is best not to smoke for your health, quite apart from the fumes making lens wear uncomfortable. You can't always avoid smoky rooms or rail compartments or buses, though, and especially at parties you are likely to find your lenses become uncomfortable. As well as cigarette fumes, the hot dryness of a crowded room will affect your eyes. Try to move away from the worst areas, and take a pair of glasses with you in case you have to change to them. If you find dry atmospheres often affect you badly, your specialist can supply eyedrops that act as artificial tears.

An irritated or infected eye   This may be due to a disorder of the lids such as a stye or blepharitis (when the lids become inflamed and flaky), or you may have an infection such as conjunctivitis. For any of these conditions you will need treatment from your eye specialist – either eyedrops or ointment. While the infection continues you should not wear contact lenses. They will prevent the condition from clearing, and at the same time they may be spoilt by absorbing germs.

During the time your eyes are sore you will have to wear glasses. This means adjusting to the different vision they give (see Chapter 2). Then when the infection or irritation has cleared you will have to go back to wearing lenses gradually, keeping them in only a few hours each day, in the same way as you became used to them when they were new. Your eyes have to adapt again to the different power of the lenses.

Make-up wrongly applied can be a cause of a lot of discomfort to contact lens wearers. You should put on eye make-up only after your lenses are in. Mascara should be used sparingly as it tends not only to enter the eye and be deposited on the contact lens, but also to impregnate the inner skin of the upper eyelid. This may even cause inflammation. Eyelashes can be dyed instead of mascara being used. You should never use liners or paints inside the lash margin as this can affect and irritate the openings of the oil secretary glands. Sometimes cosmetics themselves cause irritation and allergic reactions needing medical treatment. Obviously you should stop wearing lenses if this happens.

Some people get headaches with their lenses. You may unconsciously be holding your head in an awkward position or tensing your facial muscles because of the altered vision. Discuss this with your specialist. He or she will advise you on relaxing and holding your head properly.

A whitish discharge from the eyes is sometimes caused by contact lenses. This is due to an increase in your eye secretions, stimulated by the lenses. Use the saline eye drops recommended by your specialist, or occasionally rinse your eyes in an eye bath to wash this discharge away.

Blurring after removal of contact lenses   Sometimes blurring continues and it is difficult to see clearly with your glasses. There is more than one reason for this. If the blurring continues only for a few hours it is most likely due to lack of good breathing by the cornea. If it continues for some days after you have stopped wearing your lenses, either your glasses are no longer the right power, as your vision has changed since you began to wear lenses, or your cornea may have altered its shape. Speak to your specialist about continued blurring. Your eyes may need testing.

There are reasons why it becomes difficult to wear lenses that have more long-lasting effects. A fairly large proportion of our patients (about 25 per cent) fail to wear lenses all day after trying for three to six months. We are able to help most of them by changing their lenses or suggesting different storage solutions, but a few (10 per cent) decide lenses are not for them and go back to wearing glasses.

What are the reasons for failure?

People's sensitivity varies enormously. In general, the darker pigmented skins and eyes have better tolerance. It has been noted that people with blue eyes may be more sensitive and that fair or red-headed people may get red, sore eyes from contact lens wear.

Certainly if someone has skin trouble, especially an irritable allergic skin, contact lens wear may be a problem. Dry skin, or dandruff, can result in inflammation of the eyelids. This sensitivity often means difficulty with contact lens wear.

Similarly, people who have an allergic reaction to pollen (such as hay fever), house dust or hair, even if only at certain seasons of the year, may be badly affected by the additional problem of contact lenses and the chemical solutions that go with them.

Sometimes allergic reaction develops to the lenses themselves. It may take time to show, as it did in Alison's case:

Alison had been wearing soft lenses successfully for three years when she suddenly developed a sticky secretion and eye irritation. Slowly she found she was losing her tolerance to the lenses.

She went to see her optometrist, who could discover no change in her eyes except an inflammation of the eyelids. He realized she was getting a delayed allergic reaction to the protein coatings on her lenses and maybe to the chemicals in the lenses' storage solution as well. Gradually the chemicals had tipped the balance against Alison's tolerance.

The optometrist advised her to give up wearing her lenses for six months to allow the inflammation to die down. After that she was fitted with a new pair and now manages to avoid another reaction by having new lenses at least once a year, when her optometrist advises them. She also has to take special care with cleaning and storing her

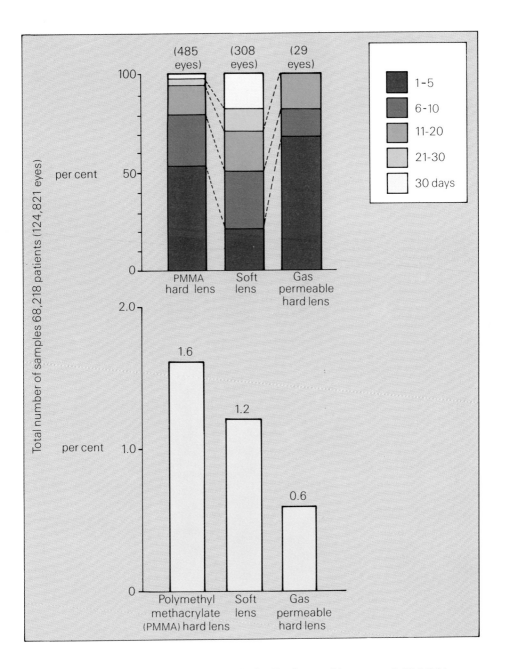

Eye injuries: these graphs from a study by Professor Hamano of 124,821 eyes show: *below*, the percentage of injury that occurred with different types of lenses, and, *above*, the average length of time for recovery. There were fewer injuries with the gas permeable type, and they healed more quickly, so if you can tolerate them, they are probably better in the long run.

lenses, avoiding solutions she knows contain the chemicals she is allergic to.

Breathing As we explained in Chapter 1, the eye needs to breathe as much as any other part of the body. Contact lens researchers have discovered that all sorts of waste products can accumulate inside the eye if it is prevented from taking in enough oxygen. They have even found that cells forming the front of the cornea will not reproduce unless the contact lens allows the eye to breathe.

Human beings can live at great extremes of temperature, from the tropical to the sub-arctic, without suffering ill effects. They can also live at any altitude from sea level to 10,000 feet (3,000 metres). Within these limits enough oxygen is supplied to the eye for contact lenses to be worn. Nevertheless, the eye tissue itself maintains in its cells very narrow limits for temperature and oxygen variations. If the environment becomes too harsh for a sensitive wearer – too hot or cold, dry, or lacking in oxygen – this may be a cause for failure.

Cry with your lenses Tears are essential for good contact lens wear. They lubricate the lens and keep the window of the eye clean and optically perfect. They are also essential for absorbing the oxygen from the air and passing it on to the eye (see Chapter 1).

When you are wearing contact lenses – especially hard ones – your eyes produce a lot of tears; you are crying because of the unusual sensation. After a few days the tearing decreases. But for the people who never adapt to hard lenses because their eyes are too sensitive, it actually increases. Excessive crying does not help since it makes the front of the eye swell very slightly and your vision becomes hazy (see Chapter 1). Nourishment is lost as the glucose from the bloodstream needed by the cornea cannot be absorbed. The lenses no longer fit well and then there is a sort of vicious circle, for the worse the fit, the less tolerant you are to the lenses.

Even with those who have adapted to their lenses there are times when the tearing comes back:

- if the lens is dirty

- or broken

- or if the wrong solution is used. For example, a soft lens soaked in a hard lens solution will produce pain and discomfort and in some cases loss of vision. As we emphasized earlier, reading the directions carefully for eyedrops, solutions or any other preparations to be used with your lenses is essential: eyes are precious.

These last reasons for crying mean temporary discomfort with your lenses and can easily be put right. If you feel this sort of discomfort, check your lenses to see if it is caused by any of them. Only if you cannot find a cause yourself will you need to see your specialist.

If you do not make sufficient tears you will not be able to wear lenses (see Chapter 1). This will be obvious very soon after you start wearing lenses. However, sometimes people develop dry eyes later in life, so that their lenses gradually become uncomfortable. A simple test your specialist may give you consists of placing thin strips of filter paper with one end just inside the lower lid and waiting for a few minutes to see how wet they become. If they become very wet you are producing enough tears; but as we have already seen it is also the quality of the tears that is important for successful lens wear and this is something that will have to be assessed at the same time.

Having a baby   Our body hormones seem to affect the quality of the tear indirectly. Some women have a feeling of dryness related to the menstrual cycle and this can also happen in pregnancy. This dryness may make contact lens wear uncomfortable and upset a successful wearer. During pregnancy women often give up wearing their lenses. Then all the extra activity involved in bringing up a small baby can relegate the lenses to the back of a drawer for good.

Taking the contraceptive pill is, from the body's point of view, like being pregnant and so some women have similar contact lens problems. One young woman remarked that she wore contact lenses because she looked more attractive without glasses but it didn't make sense to have to stop taking the pill at the same time! In our experience, however, not more than one in ten women on the pill have any dry-eye symptoms.

Illnesses such as diabetes or thyroid problems may affect your vision or the quality of the tears, so that your eyes become over-sensitive. Then it is unlikely that you will be able to tolerate contact lenses in future.

Reacting to the idea of lenses   Some people can never overcome the fear of putting something into their eye, however badly they want to wear lenses. There is nothing the specialist can do to help, and unfortunately the prospective wearer will have to admit defeat and return to wearing glasses. A few people ask if they can have surgery to correct their vision but this is often considered as a last resort and may be successful in only 70 per cent of patients.

What is the overall success rate?
Despite the initial problems and some of the long-term ones men-

tioned in this chapter, overall around 50 per cent of those who try can wear contact lenses, and in many cases people have continued for over thirty years.

Many more people are occasional users. Either they cannot get used to wearing lenses all day or they do not want to bother with constant maintenance. So they wear their lenses for short periods of four to six hours when it is important – perhaps at a party. This periodic wear is not possible, though, for most hard lens wearers, as they have discomfort with repeated insertion and removal. Even extended wear can lose its appeal, with its need for regular check-ups and renewal of lenses, and successful wearers sometimes revert to glasses.

The success rate therefore starts high – between 70 and 90 per cent – but drops rapidly after about two years of use, depending on motivation, occupation, economic and domestic problems, quite irrespective of eye tolerance.

Anyone who succeeds with contact lenses accepts a compromise. Your vision is neither the same as natural sight nor as seeing with glasses. There are the problems of tears and blurring – especially at night when the light contrast is greatest; and in Chapter 2 we explained how the image produced by lenses is different from the glasses image. Comparing one type of vision with another and expecting too much can be a reason for failure. An over-critical attitude to your contact lenses can lead to neurosis and rejection.

If you are unhappy with the results you are getting you must speak to your specialist. As long as you give a clear, accurate account of what's worrying you your specialist will be able to make the final decision as to what is best. Human error does occur and is much more likely with people who are unable to make decisions or who are unable to describe their symptoms accurately. One problem may be that your vision with contact lenses changes throughout the day. This can be improved only if you talk about it together.

If you are dissatisfied, don't act rashly, rushing to change your specialist, and then find yourself at the mercy of an unscrupulous contact lens dispenser or cleverly worded advertisement. Often all that is needed is for faith to be restored. Someone going through a phase of intolerance needs sympathy and careful assessment. Few specialists will say, 'Stop wearing your lenses for a year or two.' But a short period without them may well give you the determination to try again later.

7 SPECIAL TYPES OF CONTACT LENSES

There are now several types of special contact lenses. Some are intended to put right complex vision problems, others are cosmetic. Many are still in the early stages of development and may either not be available where you live or have not been fully approved by the profession. It is still interesting to know what is being done in this fast developing field. Yet technology moves so quickly that we can give only the information to date. No one can predict all the future types or materials or what methods of correcting vision there will be even in the next decade.

Multi-vision lenses
For anyone who is near-sighted and wears contact lenses successfully, reading becomes a problem in middle age. In Chapter 2 we explained

Multi-vision contact lenses: *left*, segment lenses, *right*, simultaneous lenses.

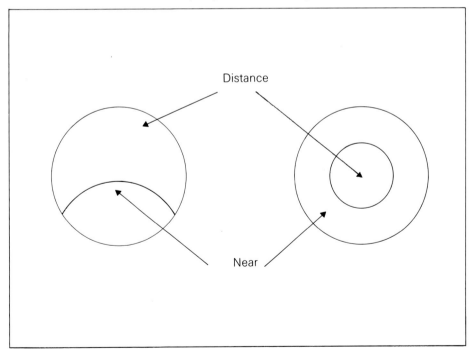

how when close vision begins to go around the age of forty (presbyopia), the problem can be overcome by wearing glasses for reading, while keeping in the lenses for distance vision all the time. Increasingly now another solution is being tried – multi-vision lenses. There are two types:

1. **Segment lenses,** generally with a lower segment for close vision and the upper for distance, like bifocal glasses. For people who have lost all close focusing there are lenses with three segments: distance, intermediate and close.

   Segment lenses work by moving upwards as the eye moves down. Since contact lenses are about 10 mm in diameter, it is difficult to use the different portions – maybe as little as 2 mm – satisfactorily.

2. **Simultaneous lenses** These have gradual (concentric) changing powers from the centre to the edge. They work without moving on the eye, but we find they are usually less effective than segment lenses.

Multifocal lenses are still not the ideal solution for near-sighted, presbyopic people. They take a lot of determination and perseverance to be useful. At present complete success is about 30 per cent for soft lenses and 40 per cent for hard.

Another way of overcoming presbyopia can be tried. One eye is corrected with a contact lens for reading and the other for distance. This may sound impossible but in practice after a few days of use many people adapt completely and are able to use the relevant lens without conscious effort.

Toric lenses
These are used for astigmatism when a simple hard lens is not successful (see Chapter 2). They are specially shaped, with non-spherical surfaces to focus the sight rays at the correct angle, and unlike the other lenses the corrective powers are normally confined to the front of the lens. A toric surface has two different curvatures at 90 degrees to each other: for example, an egg has a toric surface in any one area. A barrel too has a toric surface. Toric lenses can be kept in the correct position by being made flat below, oval in shape, or with extra thickness below (prism-shaped). They may be either hard or soft. When made of suitable materials and the right thickness they can even be used for extended wear.

If the front of the eye is astigmatic a toric lens can be used to obtain a good fit, though in practice this is rarely necessary, and because of technical difficulties in achieving the required curvature for good

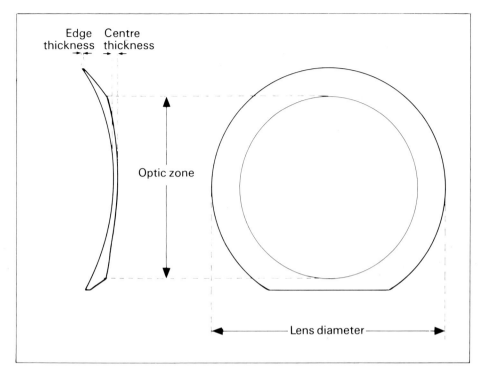

Edge   Centre
thickness thickness

Optic zone

Lens diameter

An example of a toric lens with a specially shaped surface, which corrects astigmatism by focusing the light rays at the correct angle.

vision these lenses are not commonly prescribed. When a hard contact lens has to have a toric back surface the chief problem is that the front surface must also be toric. Soft toric lenses copy the shape of an astigmatic eye and unless the front surface is made toric in the opposite direction, the vision will not be adequately corrected.

Cosmetic uses

1. Changing the eye's colour is sometimes useful for professional reasons, especially for actors and actresses. To make the eyes a different shade, either transparent, or opaque, coloured tinted contact lenses are used. A light-coloured eye can be made to look darker or even a different colour with a clear lens, but an opaque tint is needed to make a dark brown eye look, say, light blue.
   Some thick lenses have a sandwiched layer of coloured pigment that can change an eye to any colour. These are not available everywhere, however. They have yet to pass purity tests to prove that the dyes are 'fast' and do not injure human – or animal – tissue.

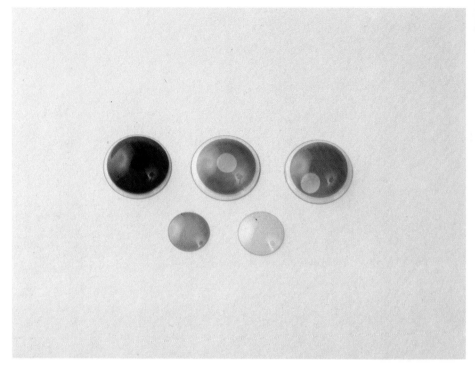

Tinted lenses used to reduce glare for people with too much light entering the eye; the lens with a darkened pupil cuts out the light altogether.

The chemical used in the colour must also be shown to agree to standards of purity.

2. Unusual or irregular-coloured eyes may be disguised with tinted lenses to give a normal appearance.

3. A deficiency of the iris that causes excessive light to enter the eye can be covered with a tinted lens.

Other uses for lenses

- Special large, flat-surfaced contact lenses help doctors in eye operations. These are placed on the eye so that internal parts such as the retina can be seen while laser or other internal eye operations are done.

- There are lenses that can be fitted with electrical terminals, and valuable information can be collected, for example:

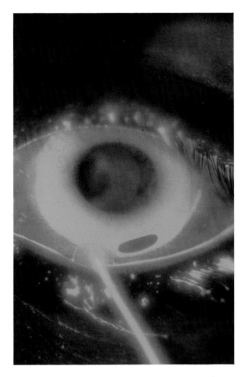
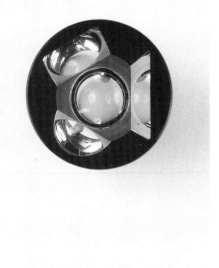

Left A diagnostic contact lens used for picking up electrical charges from the eye, and *right*, a flat lens for examining the inside front part of the eye.

1. By looking at the angle of the eye the type of glaucoma can be diagnosed
2. Foreign bodies that have entered the eye can be located
3. Electrodes fixed to the diagnostic lens pick up signals that give information about the working of the eye.

8 LENSES FOR DIFFERENT CONDITIONS

Since the introduction of contact lenses a number of eye conditions can be improved dramatically by operation and wearing contact lenses, and near perfect sight can be restored. Among these an operated cataract is probably the most successful.

Cataracts

This is a condition that occurs in many middle-aged and elderly people; the older the age group the higher the percentage of people with a cataract. About 65 per cent of men and women between fifty and sixty have one, and over sixty-five as many as 95 per cent.

The eye's lens becomes cloudy because of a change in the protein. As the cataract develops the lens becomes more and more opaque, so that vision is generally very hazy, while in bright light there is a dazzle effect. Different types of cataract can affect your vision in other ways too: if the cataract develops in the centre of the lens, it can cause double vision. With a hardening at the centre of the lens, called nuclear sclerosis, the focus is altered, causing near sight. If presbyopia was a problem before, this may even be an advantage, meaning you can do without reading glasses.

How are cataracts treated?
A lot of people do not need to have their cataracts removed. Slight blurring of the vision is not troublesome enough to make the operation worthwhile. They continue to see well enough, taking measures against the blurring and dazzle effect such as:

- Wearing a broad-brimmed hat, a shade or dark glasses in bright sunlight

- Avoiding night driving, when oncoming headlights can dazzle

- When reading, always positioning a good strong light behind the shoulder, not too far away.

Further advice for people with cataracts can be found in *Eyes: Their Problems and Treatments* by Michael Glasspool, FRCS, also in this series.

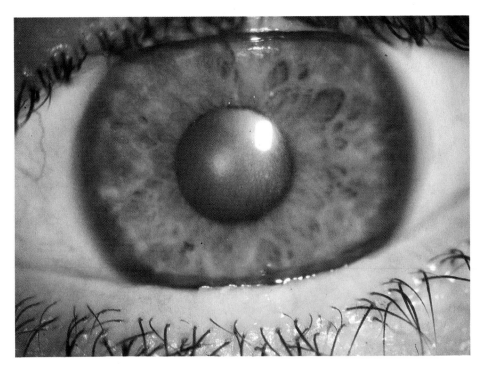
Cataract: note the clouding of the pupil area.

When the cataract is so dense that it makes everyday living difficult, it is time to have it removed. Deciding when this point has been reached rests with the eye specialist and the person concerned. The more you use your eyes for work or recreation, the clearer your sight needs to be.

The operation
For eye specialists today, this is a relatively simple operation. The cloudy lens is removed and your eye is bandaged for a few days. Once your eye is healed, you will have blurred vision and will need a replacement lens for normal focusing. Glasses, a contact lens or an implanted permanent (intraocular) lens are the options.

Glasses   These are suitable for older people who either find handling contact lenses difficult, or who would not be able to tolerate a lens implant because of another eye condition that may affect the implant.
Two pairs of glasses are needed, for near and distance vision. The disadvantage of wearing glasses after having a cataract removed is the distortion you get when looking towards the edges of the glasses lens (see also Chapter 2).

Lens implants For younger people who have had a cataract operation, this can be the ideal solution. The lens is fitted during the operation so that perfect sight is restored immediately, and there is no further trouble with putting on glasses or putting in lenses. About half the people operated for cataract have a successful lens implant. The only disadvantages are the possibilities of inflammation of the eye, or the lens moving in your eye and having to be replaced.

Contact lenses Any type of contact lens, soft, gas permeable or extended wear, may be worn after a cataract has been removed. If your eye specialist thinks a lens implant would be unsuitable for you, so long as you are able to handle them a contact lens will be prescribed. The type of lens you will be given depends on your vision and tolerance. A continuous wear soft lens is the most comfortable but it may not be adequate to correct your sight, in which case you will need supplementary spectacles or a hard, gas permeable lens of one type or another. Most people get used to this lens quickly after a cataract operation. They have the motivation, and its great advantage is that it helps the wearer to see near objects better than an implant or soft contact lens. This is because it moves more on the eye than a soft lens – and certainly than an implant, which is fixed – so that it can adjust focus better.

Getting used to contact lenses takes some time, and for older people they may be difficult to handle because of arthritic fingers, or poor remaining vision. Some people have special glasses with the lower half of the frame cut away on the cataract side. This makes seeing to handle and insert the lens easier.

Nystagmus

People with eyes that do not stay fixed but move rapidly and irregularly have the condition called nystagmus. The cause is some defect of the eye structure or nervous system from birth. Nystagmus results in poor vision as the eyes cannot stay focused on an object. Contact lenses will often help the focus better than spectacles.

Conical cornea (keratoconus)

There are several ways in which the cornea can become distorted. Sometimes people just develop a distorted cornea for no known reason. Others are due to injury. A hard blow to the eye or a burn may be the reason.

When developing from unknown causes, the cornea gradually becomes thinner than normal and pointed or conical shaped. The condition mostly affects people between the ages of twelve and twenty-five, but it is very rare. Only about one in 10,000 people develop a conical cornea, which can be treated in two ways:

- by fitting a hard contact lens
- by corneal graft.

A hard lens is fitted over the irregular shaped cornea and restores the front of the eye to its correct shape, so that light enters the eye without being distorted. This is the simpler solution and works well with people who can adapt to contact lens wear.

In Barry's case, contact lenses were the long-term solution, helping him achieve a successful career:

Barry had been at college for one year. He had left high school with good grades and was considered a first rate student. Not only was he keen on his studies but he was in the college football team. He was the only son of a couple who had married late in life. In fact, Barry's mother was thirty-six when he was born.

A hard contact lens can correct a conical cornea by restoring the original shape.

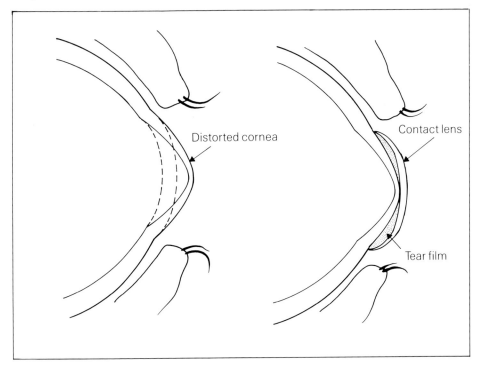

Barry noticed while writing notes in class that when he looked up the words on the blackboard were distorted. He soon found that it was only his right eye that was affected. The left was good. He blinked several times and rubbed his eyes but still the right vision was as though he was looking through a piece of cracked glass. The next few days Barry walked about opening and closing his good eye and hoping the right eye would get better, but nothing happened. He went to the medical office at the university and told the nurse about his problem. She made him read the eye chart. To his surprise, his right eye could see down to only the fourth line from the bottom while with the good eye he could easily read the bottom line. The nurse passed Barry on to the doctor, who asked him about his general health and examined his eyes with an instrument called an ophthalmoscope.

'Well, superficially the eye looks healthy,' the doctor told Barry, 'but we will get an ophthalmologist colleague to give you the once-over.'

The ophthalmologist soon found on examining the eyes with various instruments that the curvature of the cornea of Barry's eyes had become distorted and very slightly conical.

'Unfortunately glasses won't help your sight,' said the ophthalmologist, 'but I'm certain that contact lenses will.'

A small, hard corneal lens was placed in the eye and to Barry's surprise the sight improved so much he could almost read the bottom line of the chart.

Later on, after three years, the condition became a little worse with the good eye slightly affected. But with contact lenses for both eyes Barry could see almost as normal. He graduated from the university and took to a good job.

Later Barry saw the ophthalmologist again, who explained that a conical cornea (keratoconus) was a congenital weakness of the front of the eye. In most cases an operation was not necessary. Possibly children born to older mothers were more prone to abnormalities such as this. As long as they were successful, contact lenses were the best solution.

A corneal graft operation is done only if fitting the hard lens is not successful. The conical cornea is replaced with a new cornea taken from the eye of someone who has died. It is positioned with very fine nylon stitches.

Most of these operations are very successful. Since the cornea does not contain blood vessels, rejection is less likely than with other graft operations. Provided you follow the specialist's instructions and avoid any hard work or violent exercise for four to six weeks after the operation, the graft will have a chance to take successfully.

A hard contact lens may still be necessary to produce the best vision. This will be fitted several months after the operation, when it it certain that the graft has been successful and your eye will be able to tolerate the lens.

After injury for example, when an eye has been burnt with a chemical substance in an industrial accident, the skin covering the cornea may swell up, causing an irregular shaped cornea. A thin, soft hydrophilic or silicone rubber contact lens acts like a bandage. It is placed over the injured eye and allows healing to continue without irritation.

In the main part of this book we have gone into some detail about the reasons you will choose contact lenses instead of glasses, and which types are available for different vision problems. We have referred to the difficulties you are likely to find when you begin wearing lenses, and some that arise after habitual wear. In the next section is a series of questions that people frequently ask us about day to day wear.

9 QUESTIONS AND ANSWERS

We hope this section of questions often asked by wearers, and the brief replies, will be useful as easy reference. Many of the questions have probably occurred to you already. Others may not be so obvious but should be of interest and help.

What material is a contact lens made of?
The original hard lens material was PMMA (polymethyl methacrylate) but most hard materials are now mixtures of acrylate and silicone rubber so as to allow gases to flow through the material.

Soft lenses containing water mostly stem from PHEMA (poly hydroxyethyl methacrylate).

What is a cosmetic contact lens?
This is a coloured or cosmetic lens. The material is coloured to simulate a normal eye or cover areas of the eye that need protection; it can also be used to tint the light entering the eye (like sunglasses).

How long does a lens last?
It depends upon how it is used and the material. In general, constantly worn soft lenses last six months to one year, daily worn soft lenses one to two years, and hard lenses two to ten years.

What are the qualities of a successful lens?
Good vision, good tolerance, good positioning (on the centre of the eye) and no problems with the lids and eyes such as excessive redness.

Can I alternate from spectacles to contact lens wear?
If your lenses are soft, probably yes. People who find lenses difficult to tolerate often use them only for social or sporting occasions.

Can I wear contact lenses occasionally, just for parties, for example?
Rarely can this be done with hard lenses, since they need more adaptation, but with soft lenses it is possible.

Can I alternate from soft to hard lens wear?
Yes. If one sort is becoming uncomfortable your practitioner may suggest you try another for a short time.

Are there real dangers of loss of sight or even damage to the eyes and sight from contact lens wear?
The evidence of over a thirty-year period shows that the risks are small. If you are worried that your sight is getting worse, you should talk to your practitioner about it.

Do contact lenses cause allergy?
Lenses themselves will not although their protein coating may. Then, every solution does not suit everybody. Your eyes may become sensitive to a solution at any time, and if this happens you will need advice from your practitioner on changing it.

If I have to change solutions, do my lenses need adapting?
Provided the new solution is the correct type for your lenses, there is no need for this. If you follow the manufacturer's instructions it will not react with the old one.

Can children with sight defects wear contact lenses?
Yes, they tolerate lenses very well.

If an object strikes the eye will the contact lens make the injury worse?
No. In fact the lens protects the eye from extensive damage.

If my lens is damaged at the edge, can I go on wearing it?
Providing the damage is very slight, so that it neither affects your vision nor irritates you eye or eyelid, you need not replace the lens. A soft lens is less likely to irritate than a hard one when chipped.

Can a dislodged lens move behind or inside the eyeball?
No, the lens can only stay in front or under the lids.

What happens if I swallow a lens?
Nothing. The material is harmless and will pass out with bowel movement.

Do extremes of temperature and humidity such as hot or cold climates affect wear or damage the lens?
In general no, but dust, wind and excessive glare from the sun do. In dry climates supplementary artificial tear drops and more blinking are necessary.

Are contact lenses useful for extreme short sight?
Yes, better vision than with spectacles is possible.

Can they be used for long sight?
Yes, especially in the younger age groups who may also have a squint, and of course after a cataract operation.

Do contact lenses correct astigmatism?
Hard lenses certainly do and soft toric lenses correct almost 90 per cent of astigmatism.

If there is a big difference between the eyes, can contact lenses help?
Yes, the contact lens reduces the difference in vision between the eyes and enables them to work together better. So if the eyes squint (turn in or out), lenses will help correct the condition.

Do they correct colour vision defects?
Ordinary contact lenses do not help but if one lens is red and the other clear it can help reduce the problem of red-green colour blindness.

Are bifocal and trifocal contact lenses available?
Yes, but these are not always effective. Under 50 per cent of wearers find them useful.

Is there any age limit to the wearing of contact lenses?
No, providing there is someone to help with caring, putting in and taking out the lenses, there is no age limit.

Can one swim with soft water absorbent lenses?
Providing they are big enough, yes, but take them out after the swim if the water is chlorinated. Rinse in their solution and store for one hour before reinsertion.

Can one wear contact lenses during pregnancy?
Yes, but sometimes the tear secretions may change and make this more difficult.

Does everyone succeed with contact lenses?
No, only about 70 per cent over a two-year period of follow-up. We are confident the rate will improve as advances are made, but it will never be 100 per cent.

Should I feel the contact lenses even after I have adapted to their use?
In the beginning the contact lenses will be uncomfortable but when you

are fully accustomed to them you will often forget you are wearing them.

Do contact lenses fall out?
If they are fitted too loosely or if you rub your eye this can happen.
 Soft water absorbent lenses may fall out if a sharp jet of air is directed on to the eye, such as an air vent in an aircraft or car.

Should I wear lenses if my eyes are red?
Slight redness and watering often occur with hard lens wear, but if you have persistent, noticeable redness you should consult your practitioner.

If I cry, will my lenses come out of my eye?
Hard lenses may become dislodged but not soft.

Why do my lenses move over my eye?
Some movement is essential to make them function properly but the lenses should not move completely off the centre of the eye. If they do, the fit is wrong.

Can I rub my eye when wearing a contact lens?
You should massage only gently.

Can I wash my face and have a shower and/or bath when wearing contact lenses?
Certainly, providing you don't open your eyes under the water.

Can I use medically prescribed eyedrops or other eye preparations while wearing contact lenses, other than those specifically for them?
This is not advised but your practitioner will be able to give a final yes or no, depending on the medication and type of lens being worn.

Should I use eyedrops or coloured drops that I can buy over the counter or at the supermarket to soothe or whiten my eyes?
Only after asking the advice of a practitioner, since coloured drops will spoil some lenses and other drops may affect vision.

Can I use eye make-up when wearing contact lenses?
Yes, if you follow three golden rules:

1. Never use excessive make-up that is likely to enter the eye
2. Put on the make-up after inserting the lens
3. Never paint or colour the inside edge of the lid.

Can I use hair spray?
Yes, but only if you close your eyes while you use it.

I am normally a good wearer but my eye is sometimes painful after putting in a lens and even sometimes when I take one out. Why is this?
There may be a problem either with the lens or with your eye.
The lens:
- Cleaner left on the lens
- Dust, lint or deposits on the lens
- Bad or broken edge
- Crack in the lens
- Change of the lens shape
- The solution may be too strong or too weak.

The eye:
- You may have a foreign body in your eye while putting or taking out the lens
- The cornea may have an injury; you should see an eye specialist if this is suspected.

Why do my eyes become red if I read a lot or go to the movies?
If you do not blink enough when reading the lenses will become dry and your vision blurred. Then your eyes too become dry and red.

Cinemas are sometimes low in humidity and with fast moving ventilation, which also dries the eyes.

Can I sleep with my contact lenses in?
Some contact lenses are made especially for all day and night wear. Your practitioner will tell you how many days they can be worn before being taken out and cleaned. If they are not this type do not sleep in them. That can cause irritation.

Is there any difference between the left and right lens, and are they marked?
If your lenses are of different powers or fitting they may be marked with dots, letters or even numbers. Some people have their lenses faintly but differently coloured so that they never make mistakes. But there are many people who wear lenses of identical powers and fitting in both eyes, so this is not necessary.

Will wearing contact lenses feel the same all the time?
No, it is often very variable. There are good and bad days, but you should not have a progressive loss of tolerance, feeling of inflammation or weariness of the eyes. If this happens seek professional advice.

Why do I see haloes around lights and also sometimes a white flare at the fringe of my vision?
The haloes are very common with contact lens wearers. They happen at night when you are looking at lights, especially when driving a car. While they may be due to lack of 'breathing', they can also be caused by the front of the eye taking up too much water. Even with modern, thin lenses haloes may occur.

The white flare is mostly seen by people who wear hard corneal lenses and it is caused by the edge of the lens.

Can I suddenly increase my wearing time if I wear my lenses only a fixed number of hours each day?
It is better to increase the wearing time gradually. Sudden increases can cause problems.

Why is the light so dazzling with contact lenses?
This is a common complaint and indicates a reaction to the lens by the cornea. It is more common with hard lens wearers. Most contact lens wearers like to be protected from glare, sunlight and wind by wearing sunglasses.

Do I need special sunglasses to wear over my lenses?
No, any sunglasses that are comfortable and have good quality lenses are suitable.

I have to blink to see. Why can't I see clearly all the time?
If you have insufficient tears or your tears are drying up all the time, then only blinking – or using artificial tears – will keep your vision clear. If you blink and still don't see clearly the lens surface may be dirty.

Which give best sight, hard or soft contact lenses?
For simple errors of vision there is not much difference but if the front of the eye is irregular in any way (for example, owing to astigmatism) then a hard lens gives the better vision.

Why can't I see clearly if I move my eyes upwards keeping my head still?
This occurs mostly with hard or loose-fitting soft lenses, since the upper lid tends to push the lens off centre.

Why is my night vision worse than with glasses?
The contrast between light and dark objects is much greater at night and the glare and halo effect is more noticeable; this leads to less distinct images and poorer sight.

Why would I need a contact lens for an eye that has had a cataract removed?
This will restore focusing and balance the vision between the two eyes, which cannot be done with glasses.

I have had an operation to correct short sight but still require a contact lens. Why?
Many such operations do not fully correct myopia and sometimes cause astigmatism, best corrected with a contact lens.

What should I do if I spoil a lens, say by staining or grease, or it cracks or becomes misshapen?
Do not wear it and ask your practitioner for advice.

Must I always use the same preparations for cleaning my contact lenses?
Unless your practitioner says otherwise, always use the same methods and preparations.

Supposing I finish my supply of storage solution while I am away from home. What do I do?
Hard lenses can be kept temporarily in boiled tap water that has cooled. Soft lenses can be kept temporarily in distilled water that has been boiled and cooled. They should be transferred to the correct solution and left for several hours before you wear them again.

What should I do if I have soft lenses that become rough and dry while being worn?
Place them in your storage solution for a few hours and then examine them for defects.

ACKNOWLEDGEMENTS

I thank David Gifford for the drawings, Mary Banks, whose help as technical editor has been invaluable, and my wife for most of the typing and proof reading. I also acknowledge the help that the London Practice and Graham Young have given.

1985   MONTAGUE RUBEN

The publishers would like to thank the following individuals and organizations for their assistance in the preparation of this book:

For permission to reproduce photographs:

Michael Glasspool, FRCS (page 25).

The Department of Medical Illustration, Moorfield's Eye Hospital, London (pages 18, 51, 52, 69, 71).

G Nissel & Company Limited, Hemel Hempstead, photographer, David Whiting (page 39).

The photographs on the cover and pages 56-57, 58-59, 61, 66, 67, 82 and 83, right, were taken by Ray Moller, assisted by Sharon Lowery. The models are Francesca Allen, Paul Bartrop and Sarah Connearn.

The illustration on page 35 was supplied by the British Contact Lens Association.

USEFUL ADDRESSES

UNITED KINGDOM

British Contact Lens
Association
51 Strathyre Avenue
Norbury
London SW16 4RF

General Optical Council
41 Harley Street
London W1N 2DJ

Institute of Ophthalmology
41 Judd Street
London WC1 9QS

Optical Information Council
Walter House
418–22 The Strand
London WC2R 2PB

UNITED STATES

Better Vision Institute
230 Park Avenue
New York, NY 10017

Consumer Information Center
Pueblo
Connecticut 81009

Contact Lens Manufacturers
Box 1009
Mount Vernon
Ohio 43050

Myopia International Research
Foundation
415 Lexington Avenue, Rm 705
New York, NY 10017

National Association of
Optometrists and Opticians
18903 S Miles Road
Cleveland, OH 44128

National Eye Institute
Information Office
National Institute of Health
Bldg 31, Rm 6A32
Bethesda, MD 20205

National Eye Research
Foundation
18 S Michigan Avenue
Chicago, IL 60603

Public and Professional
Education Committee
American Academy of
Opthalmology
PO Box 7424
San Francisco, CA 94120

CANADA

Association of Canadian Optometrists
77 Metcalfe Street
Suite 207
Ottawa, Ontario K1P 5L6

Association of Ontario Optometrists
40 St Clair Avenue West
Toronto, Ontario
M4V 1M2

Low Vision Association of Ontario
1 Dundas Street West
PO Box 10
Toronto, Ontario
M5G 1Z3

Optometric Institute of Toronto
815 Danforth Avenue
Suite 301
Toronto, Ontario
M4J 1L2

AUSTRALIA

Australian Optometrical Association
Federal Office
2020 Drummond Street
Carlton Vic, 3053

The Optometrists' Association of NSW
234 Elizabeth Street
Sydney, NSW 2000

INDEX

Page numbers in *italic* refer to the illustrations.

Other books in the
Positive Health Guide series

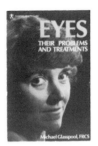

EYES
Their problems and treatments
Michael Glasspool, FRCS
Do you need glasses? How do you get rid of a stye?
What is conjunctivitis? These and many other
questions about the most common eye problems
are answered in straightforward terms by a
Consultant Ophthalmic Surgeon. There are step-
by-step instructions on everyday treatments,
putting in eyedrops, getting grit out of your eye.

Illustrated with over 30 colour and black and
white photographs and diagrams, this is the most
comprehensive book on eyes yet produced for the
layman.

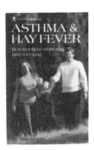

ASTHMA AND HAYFEVER
How to relieve wheezing and sneezing
Dr Allan Knight
Written by a specialist in allergies and breathing
difficulties, this practical guide shows how you can
cope with either of these common long-term
problems, suggests ways to minimize possible
irritation to a sensitive nose or lungs, includes
several easy exercises to help you relax and contains
a special section to help children prone to asthmatic
coughing and wheezing.

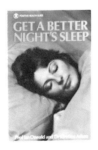

GET A BETTER NIGHT'S SLEEP
Prof Ian Oswald and Dr Kirstine Adam
For the millions of insomniacs, these world-
renowned sleep experts help to break the vicious
circle of anxiety over lost sleep leading to more
restless nights. They offer practical, scientifically
based advice on the best ways to avoid sleeplessness
and wake refreshed each morning.

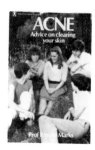

ACNE
Advice on clearing your skin
Prof Ronald Marks

A Professor of Dermatology tells you everything you need to know to help clear this condition that affects nearly all of us during the teenage years and many into their twenties and beyond.

Exploding popular myths about what causes acne, he gives practical advice on what factors to avoid, which are the most effective remedies you can buy over the counter and how you should use them. He explains how to recognize when you might need advice from your doctor and describes all the treatments he or she might prescribe.

This book will give invaluable help and reassurance both to people with acne and their parents.

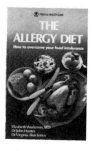

THE ALLERGY DIET
How to overcome your food intolerance
Elizabeth Workman, SRD
Dr John Hunter
Dr Virginia Alun Jones

The first recipe book presenting the famous Addenbrooke's Hospital team's step-by-step diet plan. 150 delicious recipes, over 35 illustrated in full colour, give you plenty of exciting variety while you test for the 'culprits' in your diet.

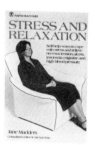

STRESS AND RELAXATION
Jane Madders

Jane Madders has developed her own simple techniques of natural relaxation that will help reduce stress in your everyday life. Tension headaches, migraine, insomnia and even nervous breakdown can often be relieved by learning to relax.

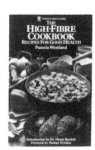

THE HIGH-FIBRE COOKBOOK
Recipes for Good Health
Pamela Westland
Introduction by Dr Denis Burkitt
Although most people now realize the enormous importance of eating high-fibre food to help avoid many of the commonest Western ailments, few know how to put this knowledge into practice in a varied and interesting way. Here at last is a book that combines the healthy benefits of high-fibre eating with good imaginative home cooking.

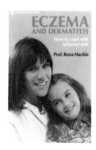

ECZEMA AND DERMATITIS
How to cope with inflamed skin
Prof Rona MacKie
Professor of Dermatology, Rona MacKie, sets out the facts about eczema in down-to-earth, reassuring terms. She gives clear guidelines on what you should do to help promote successful treatment and on what practical everyday measures you can take to avoid or at least alleviate the symptoms.

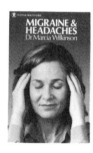

MIGRAINE & HEADACHES
Dr Marcia Wilkinson
What is a migraine? What triggers off a headache? What can you do to help yourself? Migraine clinic director Marcia Wilkinson answers these questions and many more in her reassuring guide to coping with one of the commonest, and often most distressing, medical complaints. This is an indispensable book for every migraine and headache sufferer.

BEAT HEART DISEASE!
A cardiologist explains how you can help your heart and enjoy a healthier life
Prof Risteard Mulcahy

PSORIASIS
A guide to one of the commonest skin diseases
Prof Ronald Marks

DIABETES
A practical new guide to healthy living
Dr Jim Anderson

VARICOSE VEINS
How they are treated, and what you can do to help
Prof Harold Ellis

DON'T FORGET FIBRE IN YOUR DIET
To help avoid many of our commonest diseases
Dr Denis Burkitt

THE DIABETICS' DIET BOOK
A new high-fibre eating programme
Dr Jim Mann and the Oxford Dietetic Group

THE MENOPAUSE
Coping with the change
Dr Jean Coope

OVERCOMING DYSLEXIA
A straightforward guide for families and teachers
Dr Beve Hornsby

THE DIABETICS' GET FIT BOOK
The complete home workout
Jacki Winter
Introduction by Dr Barbara Boucher

THE GLUTEN-FREE DIET BOOK
A guide to coeliac disease, dermatitis herpetiformis and gluten-free cookery
Dr Peter Rawcliffe and Ruth Rolph, SRD

THE SALT-FREE DIET BOOK
An appetizing way to help reduce high blood pressure
Dr Graham MacGregor